*Health & Longevi..,* _____ ___ _

## AYURVEDA, YOGA & NATURE CURE

For my Friend

linsy

Aman

yoqrocker@gmail.com

*Health & Longevity Through*
# AYURVEDA, YOGA & NATURE CURE

**Dr. T. L. Devaraj**

**NEW DAWN PRESS, INC.**
UK • USA • INDIA

NEW DAWN PRESS GROUP

Published by New Dawn Press Group
New Dawn Press, Inc., 244 South Randall Rd # 90, Elgin, IL 60123
e-mail: sales@newdawnpress.com

New Dawn Press, 2 Tintern Close, Slough, Berkshire, SL1-2TB, UK
e-mail: ndpuk@newdawnpress.com

New Dawn Press (An Imprint of Sterling Publishers (P) Ltd.)
A-59, Okhla Industrial Area, Phase-II, New Delhi-110020
e-mail: info@sterlingpublishers.com
www.sterlingpublishers.com

*Speaking of Ayurveda, Yoga & Nature Cure*
© 2003, Dr. T. L. Devaraj
ISBN 978-1-84557-031-6
Reprint 2005, 2008

PRINTED IN INDIA

# PREFACE

Ayurveda, an ancient science of medicine practised in India, has postulated some of the best principles for maintaining and preserving the health of any individual. It lays down certain rules, not only for healthy living, but also for hygiene – a key requisite for health.

Health is an important factor in attaining individual goals, whether it be wealth or happiness, material or spiritual, or indeed Moksha or salvation. Ayurveda stresses that the four influencing factors that play their part in gaining Moksha in the after-life are:

1. Dharma — truthful living
2. Artha — generating money and resources
3. Kama — fulfillment of desires, including the sexual
4. Moksha, itself — attainment of life's ultimate goal: Salvation

Ayurveda propounds healthy living by following a set of regimen – on a seasonal, daily and even nightly basis, coupled with sadvritta. Regimes encompass food and activity and these are detailed in this book.

The modern age is characterised by pressures – hurry, worry, the pressures of making a quick buck and the temptations of corruption. These are bound to lead to deviations from the safe routines of diet and habit, and so, to imbalances of health. The old practices of eating meals at fixed times, starting the day with exercise, supplemented with oil baths and massage, all contributed in keeping old age at bay, by keeping one's body in prime fitness, by keeping the eye keen.

However, in modern India, deviation from these principles and the effect of all manner of pollution, from food adulteration to pollution in the air and water, down to even the very lifestyles that are led, is the order of the day. Ayurveda offers relief to those suffering on account of these, whether rich or poor, in all walks of life. This book covers the ameliorating aspects of Ayurveda, for the individual and for communities. The book has four sections starting with Part A which details the historical background and basic concepts of Ayurveda before moving on to socially related issues such as Famly Planning. Ayurveda developed in order to address such community needs and this segment will examine issues of contraception and conception – such as conceiving a child of desired gender. Part B deals with topics such as the environmental perspectives of Ayurveda and issues related to the construction of communities – whether they happen to be schools, villages or cities or even just a basic lavatory. Both past and present practices are explained for the benefit of readers.

There is a special section, Part C, which is devoted to Nisargopacharam or Nature Cure, based upon the axiom of the five bhutas – air, earth, fire, water and space. These are the basic components that make up every human being, though the proportions vary from person to person. The fact is that these elements, the five bhutas, make up nature itself, Man being only a microcosm of the macrocosmic universe. This section is illustrated with photographs.

Also illustrated is the next section of the book, Part D, which deals with the subject of Yoga Vijnanam, the linkage of Yoga with Ayurveda. Postures, such as Asanas and Pranayama, which help to maintain health and can cure health problems, are explained for the benefit of the readers.

This book should prove to be valuable not only for general readers, for whom it contains matter related to the prevention of disease, protection of health and prolongation of life, but also for those students of Ayurveda who are studying for their B.A.M.S. degrees, as it covers their required curriculum.

Bangalore                                     Dr. T.L. Devaraj

# ACKNOWLEDGEMENT

I'm highly indebted to all the authors and publishers of the books quoted in the bibliography.

I am thankful to Jindal Institute of Naturopathy and Yoga, Bangalore for having permitted me to utilise the photos of Naturopathy from their publication, in this book.

I am highly beholden to Mr Govinda Rao, yoga champion of Banagiri Yoga Institute, Bangalore, for having supplied photos of yogic asanas.

I am highly obliged to Mr. S.K. Ghai, Sterling Publishers for having published this book in short time.

# CONTENTS

## Part B

## THE SCIENCE OF SOCIAL AND PERSONAL HYGIENE

### (SAMAJIKA SWASTHAVRITTA VIJNANAM
AND
VAIYUKTIKA SWASTHVRITTA)

## Part C

## NATURE CURE

### (NISARGOPACHARAM)

## Part D
### THE SCIENCE OF YOGA
(YOGA VIJNANAM)

# Part D
# THE SCIENCE OF YOGA
## YOGA VEDANTA

# PART A

## PRINCIPLES OF HEALTH AND LONGEVITY
## (SWASTHAVRITTA VIJNANAM)

# DERIVATION AND DEFINITION OF SWASTHAVRITTA

Ayurveda, is derived from two words – *Ayu* and *Veda*. **Veda** is Sanskrit for Science, while *Ayu* stands for "a beneficial life". Together they form *Ayurveda* – the science for a beneficial life. A life capable of producing happiness and health in the body, not only in this world, but also in the world hereafter.

**Swasthavritta,** is a word composed of three words, namely, *Swa, Stha* and *Vritta*. These represent three doshas in the human body, working in full cooperation and coordination with one another. Swastha itself is derived from the two Sanskrit words – **Swa** and **Stha,** and definitions in Monier William's Sanskrit dictionary for these are as follows: Swa – that which is natural, being in one's natural state, doing well, healthy in body and mind; Stha – self-abiding. Usually, " Swa " represents possession of, or, attention to, one's own.

"Stha" means one who stands, and, in the context of Ayurveda, represents stability of maintenance. In Ayurveda, only those stand and hold their own, who attach greater importance to the requirements of their bodies than they do to other attractions. **Swastha** is thus the term for a person in good health.

**Vritta** represents the existence of deliberate communication. It means "acting" or "playing one's part". In Ayurveda, it is he who acts well – such as distributing out of what he owns and discharges his bounden duties. Such a person will, sometimes, leave no stone unturned for carrying out what is proved to be beneficial by way of food and behaviour, and the rules and regimen one has to follow.

**Swasthavritta** is thus the combination of the two, and therefore the discipline that helps an individual to attain health. Health and happiness always go hand in hand, entirely interlinked; the one cannot go without the other. It is the science of Swasthavritta, which is aimed at giving happiness and a healthy and prosperous life, in order to attain Dharma, Artha and Kama in this world and Moksha in the afterlife.

**Vijnana** stands for Science or "knowledge of sciences".

## Characteristic Features of a Healthy Person

*"Samadoshah Samagnischa Samadhatumala Kriyaha Prasanna Atmendria Manaha Swastha Ityabhidheeyate!!"*

Sushrutha, one of the most well known among authorities on Ayurveda and surgery, has described the signs and symptoms of a healthy person as follows –

"The doshas must be in equilibrium and his digestive fire must be in a balanced state, while his tissues (*Dhatus* and *Malas*) must work in the normal state. The sensory and motor organs, and mind and soul (*Atma*) must also be in a pleasant state."

**Samadosha** – The Doshas which are present in the body and mind, namely the *Vata* (air), *Pitta* (fire) and *Kapha* (water), must be in a balanced state in order to keep a person healthy. If there is an imbalance, whether any of them is aggravated decreased and vitiated in any way, the state is called *Dosha Vaishamya*, a condition of diseas. These three elements, in fact, dictate and regulate the activities of even the external environment and the world, per the tenets of Ayurveda.

**Samagni** – In order to keep an individual healthy, the digestive fire – *Kosthagni*, and the tissue enzymes – *Dhatwagni* must be in their proper states. When Agni is in a depleted state, a condition known as *Mandagni*, it will be the cause of many

4

diseases. This is known as *Rogaha Sarvepi Mande Agnou* and it is well known that the health of individuals depends upon the strength of their respective digestive powers.

**Dhatus** and **Malas** – Ayurveda recognises the presence of seven substances in the body called *Dhatus*, which include the *Malas* (types of excreta). The Dhatus are – *Rasa, Rakta, Mamsa, Medas, Asthi, Majja* and *Shukra*; while the Malas are *Mala* (faeces), *Mutra* (urine) and *Sweda* (perspiration). The Dhatus and the Malas must function properly in the body for ensuring a healthy condition.

### Prasanna Atmendriya Manaha

In Ayurveda, the functions of sensory and motor organs and mind have been given special importance. When these are not in equilibrium, they will not discharge their functions properly and this will lead to the state of disease. Even when these are functioning properly, certain activities and indulgences of the body can cause them to be vitiated, again leading to a condition of disease or ailment. Ayurveda also propounds that mental health is more important than physical health; disturbances in mental equilibrium often manifest themselves physically.

Followers of Ayurveda should observe a daily regimen, from morning to evening, in addition to observing appropriate seasonal regimen for different seasons; taking care about the "where" and "how" of the construction and location of their abodes. They must learn the methods of treatment for disease produced due to the obstruction of natural urges, such as *mala* (faeces), *mutra* (urine), *kasa* (cough), *swasa* (dyspnoea), *kshawathu* (sneezing). They must learn how to prevent epidemic diseases – *Janapadadwamsa,* and to control them. They must know the rules and regulations regarding proper conduct to keep the mind at peace.

5

# HISTORICAL BACKGROUND OF SWASTHAVRITTA

Primitive people were generally very healthy, and it is only when, with the advent of "civilisation", they started to group together in towns and cities, that proliferation of disease occured. Calamities, natural and man-made; fights with animals, increase in population and the very process of migration, all contributed to injury and disease.

Ayurveda, thus, developed as both preventive medicine and as a technique of emergency treatment. In mythology, it is said, Shiva, who was the Lord of the Asuras, had vowed not to encroach upon the territories of the refined and civilised Devas, who were led by their own protector, Daksha. In spite of this vow, the Asuras continued to encroach upon more and more of the Devas' territory, leading to Daksha witholding the tribute which the Devas were supposed to give the Asuras. This act of Daksha's angered Shiva so much that he banished the Devas from their homelands and turned them into wanderers. The hardship and tribulation in the course of their wandering caused them to develop diseases such as *Gulma*, product of fatigue and malnutrition; and *Apasmara*, product of contagion. It is said that the anger of Shiva caused fevers, while unfamiliar food produced conditions such as *Prameha* and *Kushta*. Mental disturbance, stress and anguish at the loss of loved ones and property, caused *Unmada*. Shiva's own excited mental state produced a condition known as *Raktapitta*, and esoteric acts such as the excessive sexual activity of the Moon God, the King of the Nakshatras, introduced consumption. Disease was now rampant among the Devas, and, desperate for solutions, they appointed the Ashvani Kumaras for seeking remedies. *Accordingly, it was the Ashvani Kumaras who obliged; performing wonders such as rejoining the head of Daksha to its body after he had been beheaded by the Asuras, then curing Indra of his paralysis and finally, the Moon God of his consumption. The aged Chyavan Rishi was rejuvenated and became young once again, with complete restoration of his sexual prowess.*

Based on popular demand, the Ashvani Kumaras developed a science for the preservation of health and sent the learned Bharadwaja Muni to teach the Rishis for the propagation of this science. Meanwhile, they explored and learned the principles of longevity and continued to investigate general rules of diagnosis and treatment.

These included prophylactic techniques, substances with medicinal properties, and special cases and exceptional treatments. This earned them renown, and among them, Punarvasu imparted his highly developed knowledge of Ayurveda for maintaining good health, to six of his disciples with the mission of propagating this science to the humans on Earth. While each of the six wrote individual treatises, one in particular is very well known and highly relevant even in modern times. This is Agnivesha's treatise, which he called **"Agnivesha Samhita "**.

# THE PHYSICALLY PERFECT
# HUMAN BODY

The living human body consists of the physical body with its various organs, mind and soul. A human body can be recognised as healthy from the condition of its constituents, the solidarity and healthy condition of its *Twak* (skin), *Mamsa* (muscle and tissue), *Medas* (fat), *Asthi* (bones), *Majja* (marrow), *Sukra* (semen), and last but not least, Character. The physical body is a function of the relative proportions of body parts, the influence of available food stuff, the amount of food intake, the mental aspect and the ability to work with ease.

## Visible Physical Characteristics

Some of the visible physical characteristics indicative of a perfect specimen are – the forehead must be prominent, with its lower end near the ears also so. The hair on the body should grow from one stem and be smooth, soft, fine and be well attached to the skin. Ears should appear small when seen from in front, but must be large, raised and fleshy. The eyes should show both the black and white parts clearly; eye lashes thick and well-set. The nose should be straight and moderately prominent, fleshy, with nostrils slightly flared. Lips must appear red and should not protrude. Jaws should be large but not prominent, and the mouth should be big, with uniform, glossy white, smooth, well-set teeth. The chin fleshy. The neck should be long and rounded. The abdomen should be slightly prominent with a depressed navel. Nails should be red, thin and convex in shape, set in hands and feet that are fleshy, big, glossy and tinged reddish. Fingers should be long, without spaces in between. The back should have a layer of flesh, and expansile joints, strong and fleshy. Skin colour should show gloss and life, be smooth and pleasing to the eye, perhaps with a covering of soft down. The voice should be loud and clear, perhaps with a nasal twang. The body should exhibit strength naturally – a strength that is enduring. To be considered healthy, the body should not have suffered from disease from childhood, properly grown in stature, as well as in its mental faculty. These happen to be the conditions that ensure requisite health and wealth for its owner. Happiness, fortune and authority can be considered natural for such an individual.

The presence of the normal and desired amount of **Rakta** in an individual leads to a reddish complexion and gloss, especially in the eyes, ears, mouth, nose, lips, tongue, soles, palms, nails, generative organs and forehead. Such individuals are expected to have happiness, self-respect, high intelligence, exhibit tenderness and to be able to face difficulty with equanimity. When **Mamsa** is present in an individual in the normal and desired amount, his forehead, eye, back of neck, chin, stomach, armpits, shoulder, breasts and the joints of the face and hands will appear solid, attractive, heavy and well muscled. Such an individual will have a tendency towards forgiveness, steadiness, fortitude, pleasantness, health, strength and long life. When **Medas** (fat) is present in an individual in normal and desired amount, then his heels, ankles, knees, collar bone, elbows, chin, teeth and forehead will be large and the person will be able to bear hardships, have the ability to withstand even unusual amounts of tension and adverse environment both mentally and physically, and be able to carry out great works with enthusiasm and vitality.

Such a being will live long. The presence of the ideal amount of **Majja** (marrow) will result in the individual having glossy skin, big, long and rounded joints, a soft but strong body. It foretells strength, both mental and physical, wealth, fecundity and a scholarly disposition and assures an honourable social status. The presence of the ideal amount of **Shukra** (semen) will result in the individual having an affectionate demeanour, mild and joyful in temperament. It will cause his hair and teeth to be strong, rounded, uniform and glossy, and his voice and skin tones to be pleasing. His hips will be large and strong and so will be his sexual appetites. In addition to health, wealth and happiness, he will breed prolifically.

An individual of ideal character will exhibit good manners, always doing good things, exhibiting wisdom, gratitude and virtuousness. Pure in heart, extremely sincere and attentive about his duties, such a person will be careful about serving others as well as himself. He will be brave, valiant and firm; not one to yield to disappointment and rejection. He will have great patience and will earn high respect in society. He will be innovative about the way he does things. Individuals who possess the ideal attributes of the physique and mind, much as has been outlined above, will be very strong and go on to enjoy the pleasures of this world while living long and happily.

**Proportions of the Ideal Body**
The ancient sages used parts of the human body itself for their measurements. As given in Charaka Samhita (Charaka's treatise) and Sushrutha, the circumference of one's own middle finger is called an **Amguli** or **Amgula** and used thereafter for purposes of measuring.

The ideal height for a man should be 84 amguli, while his shanks should be 40 amgulis long and 16 in girth. His knees should be 4 amgulis long and 16 in girth; his thighs should be 18 amgulis long and 30 in girth; his testes should be 5 amgulis long and 8 in girth; and his generative organs should be 6 amgulis long and 5 in girth. For the female, the generative organs should be 12 in girth. The waist should be 16 amgulis in width, the stomach 10 amgulis in width and 12 in length, and the region of the ribs, 10 amgulis in width and 12 in length. The circumference of each areola of the nipples should be 2 amguli. The distance between two shoulders should measure 24 amguli when expanded and be 12 amgulis in height. The breadth of the heart, shoulders and chest should be 2, 8, and 5 respectively. The neck should be 4 amgulis in height and 22 in circumference, while the face, including the mouth, should be 12 amgulis in height and 24 in circumference. The mouth itself should measure 5 amgulis, while each of the chin, lips, ears, eyes and the centre part of the nose and forehead should be of 4 amgulis. The head itself should be 16 amgulis long and 32 in circumference while the whole body itself should be 84 amgulis long.

**Measurements of the Ideal Body According to Sushrutha–** Sushrutha adopted the **Hasta** in addition to the amguli as his units of measurement. The Hasta is derived from the amguli and 24 amguli are equal to one Hasta. According to him, although the height of the man may be as much as 120 amgulis, in order to live happily, a person should be 3½ hasta tall, taking one's own hasta as the measure. Also, according to him, the primary parts of the body are the trunk, the superior extremities, the head, the toe and the second digit of each foot. The toes and this digit should each be of 2 amgulis in length. The third, fourth and fifth digits of the foot should be progressively 1/5 less in length.

The parts which are of only 2 amgulis in size are the chin, testes, teeth, each side of the nose, the root of the ears, inner portions of the eyes, the distance between two pupils, and the penis when flaccid.

The breadth of the mouth should be 4 amgulis and the circumference 20 amgulis while the nostrils should be 1½ amgulis. And the circumference of the cornea should be 1/3$^{rd}$ that of the eyes.

The circumference of the pupil should be 1/9$^{th}$ that of the cornea. The hairline should be 11 amgulis from the centre of the top of the head, while the occipital protuberances should be 10 amgulis away. The index and the fourth finger should measure 4½ amgulis, the thumb and the little finger should measure 3½ amgulis. The distance between the root of the thumb and the index finger, the distance between the ear and the lateral angle, and each of the two middle fingers should measure 5 amgulis.

The forefoot and the arch of the foot should be 5 amgulis in length and 4 in breadth, and the circumferences of each of the feet, ankles, calves and knees should be 14 at their centres. The calves should be 18 amgulis long, the length from hip to knee joint 22. The length of the thigh should be equal to the length of the leg and of 12 amgulis. The length of the perinium, from the tip of the coccyx to the symphysis pubis, the distance between the penis umbilicus, the umbilicus to the heart, the heart to the root of the neck, the distance between the two breasts, the length of the face – from tip of chin to the upper border of the forehead, and finally the the circumference of wrist and elbow should all measure 12 amgulias. The distance from mastoid tuberosities from behind should be 14 amgulias. The circumference, at the centre of the calf, of indrabasti and the length between the top of the shoulder and the elbow should be 16 amgulis. The woman's buttocks or pelvic region should have the same proportions as the chest of a man, while her chest should be 18 amgulis in breadth and equal to the measurements of the male pelvic region.

The hasta of 24 amgulis also corresponds to the length from the elbow to the tip of the middle finger. The distance between the hip and any of the shoulders should be 32 amgulis. The distance between wrist and elbows should be 16 amgulis. The length and breadth of the palms of the hand should be 6 and 4 amgulis respectively. The man or woman with these ideal proportions is expected to be blessed with good health and wealth.

## Influence of Food Substances

Generally, a man who is accustomed to take food with six **Rasas**, or flavours, will have a long and blissful life. Those who are in the habit of imbibing an abundance of milk, cream, ghee, oil, meat along with other hard substances, are in danger of facing hardship.

## Food Intake

When nutritious food is consumed, it will be digested easily. The consumer of such food will adjust to climatic changes and such a person may quite easily live to a hundred years.

## The Mental Aspect

The mind is controlled by the body, and the **Atma** inside it regulates all the functions of the body – the outstanding, the ordinary and the evil. Those with outstanding minds will be of good character and have the ability to face the hardships of life, while those with commonplace minds are liable to end up in hard circumstances. An ideal body, when fit, can produce much work even when it is aged.

People with bad and evil tendencies cannot stand up to adverse circumstances. Even with good physiques, such people are prone to being carried away by sentiment and find difficulty in bearing pain and disappointment. As an example, even the sight of blood triggers loss of control or fainting fits in such. They may not be relied upon for any work.

# DAILY DUTIES AND HEALTH

Daily duties play a major role in the regulation of not only the body but also the mind. Ayurveda advocates that a healthy person must rise from his bed early in the morning, about three hours before sunrise and perform important morning ablutions, such as evacuating his bladder and bowel without inhibiting them.

He should clean his teeth with one of the parts of any of the trees mentioned – *Arka, Kadira, Nyagrodha, Karanja, Kakubha* or *Nimba*. Before these plant parts are used, they must be cleaned thoroughly and made into a brush-like form before actually rubbing them on the teeth. The rubbing action should be gentle, so as not to harm the gums. However, the actual choice of tree whose part is taken is determined by the individual constitution of the user, the mix of Doshas in his or her body determining the choice of tree, the causes of odour in the mouth and improve the person's feeling of well being.

Once the tongue has been cleansed, a gargle with the proper oil is called for. The fluid should be held for some time in the mouth to allow it to soak in to enhance its benefits. This is good for the teeth and will make them strong and hard and minimise the chances of disorders of the mouth during a person's lifetime. Besides this, it will also strengthen his chin and voice, and improve his taste for food.

**Benefits of Gargling** – Gargling increases digestive power, purifies the stomach, leading to an improvement in physical strength and a brightening of the colour of the eyes. It increases the activities of the organs. It prevents old age and extends life – to a century and more.

A person should wash his face and eyes with cold water, or preferably, with a decoction of **Triphala**. Using the decoction of tree barks in a base of milky juice cleans the face and prevents dryness of the mouth, while preventing **Raktapitta** (haemorrhagic disorders). Such decoctions are good for the complexion, as well as enhancers for eyesight.

**Benefits of Applying Kaajal** – Antimony collyrium should be applied on a daily basis, to the eyelashes as well as to the eyes directly. Rasanjanas are also to be applied once or twice a week in order to remove tears and sticky matter from the eyes, and especially for disorders of Kapha Dosha. The benefits of applying collyrium to the eyes may be listed as follows:
1. alleviates itching and burning sensations
2. removes dirty secretion
3. stops the eye from watering
4. protects against infection
5. improves / enhances appearance
6. improves ability to see in conditions of stiff breeze or bright sunshine

The actual process of applying collyrium should not be done by day, but rather two and a half hours before sunrise.

Collyrium is prohibited, in the following situations (as it weakens the eyes):
- if a person has already taken food
- if a person has already taken a head bath
- if a person is in a fatigued condition due to intense physical exercise
- after a sleepless night vigil

**Preparation of Anutaila** – Another application is that of oil in the nostrils. This is called **Nasya** (Errhine). *Anutaila* is usually used for this purpose and can be prepared by taking an equal measure of the drugs *Chandana, Agaru, Pata, Darvi, Tuwaraka, Madhuka, Prapundreeka, Sukshamaela, Vidanga, Bilva, Utpala, Hrivera, Abhaya, Vanya, Musta, Sariva, Jeevanti, Shatavari, Padma, Kesara, Surabi, Vyagri, Brihati* and such. These are first mixed, after which, exactly hundred times their weight in water is added to the mixture. This is then boiled, until the volume reduces to a tenth of the original. The wet mix is now divided into 13 parts and an equal quantity of oil is added before boiling again, until the water completely evaporates. This is repeated nine times by adding water and boiling it to evaporation. Finally, an equal quantity of sheep's milk is added and boiled one last time, till all fluid has evaporated. This preparation

**Applying Anutaila** – 5 to 10 drops of Anutaila should be placed in the nostrils, in the mornings during the Sharad and Vasanta seasons, around noon during the cold season, and in the evening in the hot season. During the rains, it should be applied when the sun is out.

**Benefits of Anutaila** – This regime imparts the following benefits:

1. The eyes, nose and ears continue to function normally throughout life.
2. Prevents graying of hair and hair loss.
3. It is the cure for diseases such as *Manyasthamba, Shirashula* (headache), *Ardita* (facial paralysis), *Peenasa* (rhinorrhea), *Ardhavabhedaka* (hemicrania) and *Shirakampa* (cerebral palsy).
4. It keeps blood vessels, joints and muscles strong.
5. It improves appearance and voice.

6. Maintains the functioning of all the organs of the head, while protecting against diseases of the head and the rest of the body. Arrests aging of the head even in old age.

**Errhine Therapy** – The patient's head must be given an oil massage and exposed to Sweda, that is, made to sweat. Caution should be exercised to ensure that sweat does not get into his eyes and cause irritation or interfere with vision. The patient should lie on a bed, in an unexposed place, free from currents of external air. Anutaila is then soaked into a piece of cotton wool and squeezed into one nostril, while keeping the other closed. After both nostrils have been given their dose, the palms of the hands, soles of the feet, shoulders and ears must also be massaged with oil. After holding his reclining position for a minute or two, to allow the decoction to soak in, the patient must then gargle with hot water to remove oily residues and the Kapha present in the mouth. Finally, the patient has to take in a bout of medicinal smoking to protect his head against the vitiation of Kapha and Vata.

**Medicated Smoking (Dhumrapana)** – Medicated smoking is indicated in the following cases:
- Hoarseness of voice
- Malodour in the nose and mouth, and nasal disease
- Paleness of face
- Hemicrania
- Hiccups
- Weakness of teeth
- Distaste for food
- Stiffness of neck, the joints and skin
- Wet and dry types of Kapha
- Malfunction of intelligence
- Tendency for excessive sleep

**Types of Dhumrapana** – Dhumrapana or medicated smoking is of three classes – *Snigdha* (pacifying), *Madhyama* (moderately exciting) and *Teekshana* (exciting).

The first two categories of medicated smoking are used for curing conditions involving Vata and Kapha. The Teekshana type is used for people suffering from diabetes, dropsy, loss of sight, Adhmana, Rohini, anaemia, head injuries, Urdhvavata, indigestion, delirium, insomnia and dryness of the palate. It is also performed after enema therapy, eating meals involving fish, wine, milk, curd, honey, and oil. It also benefits pregnant women. The dose for the Snigdha variety is just once per day, following expression to natural urges, such as after passing motion or urine, sneezing, yawning, sex, cleaning teeth and shaving. The Madhyama, twice a day, once after food and then per the regime outlined for the Snigdha. Teekshana, must be given three to four times a day, after sleep, nasya, anjana, bathing or emesis.

However, it must be borne in mind that untimely or excessive Dhumrapana can lead to loss of sight, Raktapitta, loss of consciousness, excessive thirst, madness, deafness and insensibility.

**Apparatus for Dhumrapana** – The pipe that is to be used for smoking should be made of metal and be divided into three compartments. The outlet holes for these compartments should not face each other. While the pipe should be straight in shape, one end should be slightly larger, about ¾ inch, than the other. The length of the pipe should vary depending upon the type of smoking and be 32 amgulis for Snigdha Dhumrapana, 42 amgulis for Madhyama Dhumrapana and 24 amgulis for Teekshana Dhumrapana.

**Preparing a Medicinal Wick** – A grass stick, 12 amgulis in length is taken, soaked in water for 24 hours before it is removed and coated with the medicinal pulp which is described below. This coating may be required to be applied about five times before it is of the size that will fit inside the diameter of the pipe. The wick is now set to dry out in the shade. When required for actual use, the wick is first rubbed with oil.

The medicinal pulp used for Snigdha Dhumrapana may utilise some of the following: *Agaru, Guggulu, Usira, Mustha, Madhuka, Madana, Vasa, Yava, Kumkuma, Kaunti, Elavaluka, Srivetaka, Sararasa, Sthouneya, Tila* and oils, such as ghee and those derived from fruits.

The medicinal pulp used for Madhyama Dhumrapana may utilise: *Ashvatta, Udumbara, Laksha, Prithvika, Kamala, Nyagrodha,* the bark of *Plaksha, Padma, Raktavesti, Kusta, Tagara, Yastimadhu* and sugar.

The medicinal pulp used for Teekshna Dhumrapana may utilise:
*Laksha, Triphala, Jyotishmati, Nisha, Swetha, Vidanga* and *Tagara.*

Dhumrapana is basically inhaling smoke through the nose and then exhaling it through the mouth, and the basic technique should be so maintained. The body posture of the smoker should be kept straight, with the mind concentrating on the technique. The mouth should be kept open to facilitate exhaling. This is important because exhaling through the nose is likely to lead to the smoke getting to the eyes and affecting them injuriously. However, the technique does vary, depending on where the doshas causing the particular affliction happen to be located. If the vitiated doshas are in the nose and head, it becomes standard practise to inhale through the nose. On the other hand, if the vitiated doshas happen to be in the throat, inhalation should be done from the mouth.

**Tambula** – is prepared as a mixture containing Camphor, *Katuka, Trikatu,* ginger, both black and long pepper, lime and betelnut powder, wrapped in a betelnut leaf. When ingested, this removes dirty excreta from the teeth and mouth, strengthens heart functions and alleviates nausea. However, it is contraindicated in the case of the following conditions:

Raktapitta, wounds in the mouth, exhaustion, fainting fits, thirst, dryness of the mouth, loss of weight, weakness and effects of poisoning, such as insensibility and defective vision. The betel-leaf must be chewed and masticated thoroughly in the mouth, until nothing is left, in order to make the most of it.

**Abhyanga Oil Massage** – A special oil called *Abhyanga* is used for this massage and the benefits derived include the easing of disorders of the Kapha and Vata, cleansing of the skin and the body, soothing muscles, better sleep due to the relaxing effects, improving eyesight, banishing exhaustion and improving skin tone. Application of the oil on the head, ears and feet will prevent and ameliorate headaches.

*Chakratail* was the base for the oil, advocated by Sushrutha, for the Abhyanga of the head. Some drugs which are mixed into the massage oil are *Devadaru, Sarala, Madhuka* and *Kshudraka.*

The ears can become afflicted owing to vitiation of Vata and applying this oil on a daily basis will prevent any ear disease, as well as providing protection against stiffness of the chin and the neck. This will also improve the ability of withstanding loud noises and prevent deafness and headache. It will also remove grime and germs from the ears and improve the all-round quality of hair. In fact, it will provide benefit to all symptoms of the vitiation of Vata, such as cracks in the foot, formation of callus, roughness, tiredness, lack of neural feeling and problems with sight. It will contribute to proper sleep rhythms and will act as an aphrodisiac.

Two additional methods of Abhyanga propounded by Shushrutha are *Pariksheka*, the sprinkling type and *Avagha*.

**Pariksheka** – A mixture of suitable oils is prepared and is poured continuously, from a distance of 13 amgulis on the body (when that part is being treated) or, from a distance of 4 amgulis on the head. This provides synergy to the process of removing vitiated Vata. Synergy to alleviating exhaustion and exertion, to providing strength to the heart, to healing broken bones, wounds, burns, scratches and all manner of injury. An extension to this technique is to make the patient sit, partly immersed, in a tub of oil. However, it should not be used after an administration of purgatives or emetics or when the patient has suffered a bout of indigestion or fever, or those suffering from diseases resulting from obesity.

However, there is such a thing as excessive exercise and some of the adverse effects may be severe weight loss, distaste for food, nausea and vomiting, haemorrhagic disorders, delirium, exhaustion, anaemia and fever. Exercise is contraindicated in the case of people suffering from vitiation of Vata, Pitta, Doshas and indigestion. Also, in the case of those in a state of exhaustion, those who may be promiscuous, the constant traveller, the overworked and the fatigued, and those who have either just taken a meal or those who are hungry or thirsty.

Hard exercise demands being strong in the first place, so good nutrition is a must. The weather is also a determinant, cooler times and seasons, such as Vasanta Ritu being preferred.

**Mardhana** (Massage) – Of the many massage techniques employed in Ayurveda, the three most important are *Udvartana, Udgarshana* and *Utsadana*. **Udvartana** is the act of a rubdown with ointment after a bout of exercise. By removing perspiration, it removes fat and the vitiated Kapha and Vata Doshas. It is good for strength and skin tone.

**Udgarshana** and **Utsadana** are more vigorous massages and the former, where a brick is used, is meant only for males, and when coupled with Udvartana, will help in the expansion and dilation of blood vessels and provide warmth to the parts where applied to. It may also be employed for cases of itching and ring-worm. Utsadana, is exclusive for females.

21

**Snana** (Bath) – After exercise it is essential to bathe, and the benefits of this act of cleansing cannot be over-emphasised. Bathing contributes to improvement in digestive power, lengthens life, physical strength and sexual enthusiasm, removes itching, burning sensations and exhaustion, removes sweat, imparts alertness and a feeling of lightness. It regulates every part of the body to work with zeal and enthusiasm, besides purifying blood and imparting a pleasant feeling. However, there are some cases for not bathing and these could include diarrhoea, fever, distension, indigestion, distaste for food, eye, mouth and hair diseases and just after a meal.

Hot water is indicated during the cold season and whenever there is a disease of the Vata and Kapha, which produce haemorrhagic disorders. Cold water has a tendency to increase Vata and Kapha related conditions. It is preferable to use hot water for the body but cold water for the head.

This provides strength to the head and to the lower part of the body, while keeping the eyes and hair in good condition.

**Apparel** – Ayurveda advocates wearing clean garments, banishing the unpleasant from personal life, and the use of deodorant to enhance the feel of a clean body and to control body odours. Following this principle, improves not only hygiene, but also peace of mind; prerequisites for longevity. Use of perfumes will, quite obviously, also improve sexual attraction. Ayurveda also recommends wearing shoes, a turban on the head, carrying an umbrella and a strong stick for walking outdoors.

**Ornaments and Applications** – Ornaments, suitably selected and worn, are believed to bring good fortune and a long life. Ayurveda has also developed cooling salves for the face, which when applied, are believed to contribute to beauty, eyesight and remove skin defects, besides making one feel fresh. Mainly for the fairer sex, Ayurveda recommends the application of cosmetics such as collyrium, to the eyelashes in order to keep them in a good condition and to enhance brightness and clarity of vision, besides enhancing beauty.

**Worship** – Worship of God is a core neccessity for followers of Ayurveda, essential for ensuring success in life, as well as longevity. Worship of God is considered the first among sixteen daily duties advocated. The others include even such mundane acts as shaving, combing and grooming. Such simple acts are pleasurable in themselves while promoting a sense of well being. The old practitioners recommended that these were to be the first acts of the day for any individual, starting three hours before sunrise. The feeling of well being thus obtained would then last through the day.

**Walking** – Walking is one of the easiest ways to keep the body in prime condition. The more one walks, the better, stopping as fatigue sets in, for a good rest for the body and the mind. Walking is good for strength, memory, stamina and digestion.

**Food** – Ayurveda propounds that food must be taken in moderate quantities and only after the previous meal has been fully digested.

It cautions against overeating. The food must be pleasant in taste and should be pure, fresh and moderately warm. It should not burn the mouth. Sweets are supposed to be eaten first, followed by the sour and the salty and other tastes at the end. Vegetables with fibre content are recommended towards the first half of the meal. During the meal, the person who is eating, should sit straight, with the mind focussed on the meal, excluding distracting thoughts and worries during the meal. The meal finishes with drinking plenty of liquids. Warm food is conducive to quick and easy digestion. When nights are short, the first main meal is recommended for the afternoon and the second at night. Before any food is taken, the mouth should be washed with pure and clean water. This prevents the ingestion of stale matter and improves taste for the preparations that will follow. Sweet foods impart energy, pleasantness, enthusiasm, nourishment and appetite. It is essential to wash the mouth at the conclusion of all meals. As soon as food is ingested, the Kapha levels increase and during digestion the Vata levels increase. Dhumrapana and taking Tambula containing astringent, pungent and bitter substances is recommended. Finally, one should rest after the meal.

**Occupational Activity** – Rest and recreation after a period of occupational activity are important components of life, per Ayurvedic tenets. It is the duty of every individual to earn money in order to live life happily and healthily, and one should engage in occupational work, followed by rest and recreation between one meal to the next. Sleep should follow as a feeling of having had adequate recreation sets in.

**Meditation** – Meditation is considered a daily essential, and recommended for the few moments just before sleep. Meditation, at the very basic level, may consist of being as simple as recapitulating how the day was spent, tinged with judging oneself for one's activities and performance. These sessions can become a source of contentment through life.

**Sleep** – Sleeping at night is a healthy practise for both body and mind. One must go to bed early.

# 5

# SLEEP AND HEALTH

Natural sleep at night is essential for health, human rhythms being naturally attuned to that of the Earth's. Humans produce *Tamoguna* while awake and this shortens lifespan.

**Charaka's Sutra regarding Sleep** – In Chapter 21 of his Charaka Sutra, the great sage Charaka dealt with the benefits and the not-so-beneficial aspects of sleep. He stated that with proper sleep one derives happiness and an increase in lifespan. Practitioners of Yoga can control their sleep to derive benefits of intellect, truth, activeness, good digestive systems and to balance their dhatus. Sleep is as much a requirement as food and the night is the time to get it. There is a vitiation of Kapha levels and alleviation in Vata and Pitta levels in the human body, leading to strength and robustness. Seven benefits listed by him are:
- Happiness
- Robustness
- Strength
- Virility
- Power
- Knowledge
- Longevity

However, sleeping at odd hours can make the sleeper prone to any of the following – giddiness, fever, unhappiness, **Sthaimitya** (feeling cold), rhinorrhoea, headache, grief and

25

indigestion. This has been reinforced by Sushrutha, in Chapter 4 of his treatise "**Shareera**", where he has stated that proper sleep fortifies the immune system and keeps disease at bay. Also, that it gives clarity of mind, strength, virility, adds colour to life and helps in proper balancing of the weight of an individual. He felt that sleep brought about the blessings of Lakshmi, thus attracting riches and that regular sleepers lived beyond an age of a hundred years.

**Sleep and Health**

Sleeping during the day is likely to render the body 'unctuous' by day, although he made an exception in the case of married couples and for the summer season.

For those with a problem of excessive sleeping, he recommended purgatives, errhines, emetics, meditation and stimulation of thinking, imposition of scary situations or sleeping in an uncomfortable bed, exercise, blood letting and fasting. Vitiation of Vata leads to such a condition and to overcome it one has to develop Satvaguna, courage and practise concentration on work.

A good night's sleep is natural for those practising Brahmacharya and those fortunate enough in having opportunities for *Gramya Dharma* (coitus) and mental peace. Sleep, food and Brahmacharya are considered to be the three pillars for maintaining the health of any individual.

# 6

# SEX AND HEALTH

The balance of the physical body is completely dependant upon its activities, especially the effects that its sexual activity creates and the mental attitude of the person involved. In the olden days, and even till the nineteenth century, life itself was very uncertain. This called for having large families, to provide for an adequate workforce for agriculture or industry and to account for attrition by way of early mortalities. So, many progeny were necessary and having many, generally meant a better status in society.

As population increased, the need for many progeny declined and correspondingly, the average numbers of children in any family fell, from ten to eight, to five and so on, until the present day, when families with a single child are common. The sexual act, in addition to being meant for the production of progeny, has on the other hand, assumed the dimensions of an act of enjoyment. This appears to also have been the case during Charaka's times, characterised by lusty people, although the female of those times was generally, just a passive dummy. So, sexual health, during his times, was as important a consideration, as it is today. All living beings desire sex, for pleasure, as well as, to continue the line.

Nature has the onerous duty to continue the species and this is one of three obligations that are to be discharged by all men; the other two being discharge of debt and achieving prosperity. Debt includes that which we owe to the Rishis (learned men, sages and great teachers) and the Devas (supernatural beings with superpowers). Accordingly, Charaka had advocated the concept of lawful marriage for the sake of progeny. This allowed one the freedom of selecting a partner, based on individual preference. After all, relations between husband and wife after marriage are only likely to be effective when both partners are pleased with the other. Not having an issue being a basic cause for dissatisfaction.

**Sex and Health**
His prescription for marital status – as relevant now as it was then – is that one's partner should be legally wedded to one and in perfect health.

He emphasised that coitus be performed in a way, and at a place, that does not cause inconvenience to either partner. He recognised concepts such as that of a beloved – a partner in every sense - one that is attractive to the other and who enjoys the fullest confidence and trust of the other. Cautioning against sexual overindulgence and promiscuity, stating that this led to consumption and even death, he maintained that sex, if used with caution, will not only support the body as a pillar does the house, but that it is simultaneously a great provider of mental stimulation and satisfaction. He advocated the use of aphrodisiacs and allowed for the effect of the seasons, allowing sexual activity to capacity in the cold weather, but tempered with three day abstinence during the Vasanta and Sharad seasons and once in fifteen days during all others. He warned of the complications of excessive coitus, such as, drooping of the thighs, langour and lassitude, loss of physical strength, loss of dhatus and tissue and minerals, and finally, atrophy l containing sugar and meat, drinks containing the juice of pulses, wine or water and finally sound sleep. According to its tenets, a man can perform coitus with a married woman only after her sixteenth year and till the time he reaches seventy. The Dharamashastras have opined that it is only natural for humans to want to have sexual relations with the opposite sex for deriving sexual happiness, and so no blame can be attached to such urges. However, the same Shastra then insist on a level of continence after achieving Grihasthashrama and Vanaprathasthashrama, when a vow should be taken for celibacy. Hereon, the individual must concentrate on more efforts at earning, giving up all interest in any position and sleeping on the bare ground if required.

# 7

# SEASONAL CONDUCT AND HEALTH

There are six seasons, called *Ritus*, in a year and each season lasts for two months approximately, completing the yearly cycle in twelve month. The year begins with the season of *Sisira*, followed by *Vasanta, Greeshma, Varsha, Sharad* and *Hemanta*. Ayurveda has divided the year into two principal parts, namely, *Uttarayana*, starting with Sisir and ending with Greeshma, and *Dakshinayana*, starting with Varsha and ending with Hemanta. Uttarayana, is the period of increasing heat and ennervation, while Dakshinayana is the period of increasing cold and energy. The produce that is available for human consumption accordingly differs from one part to the other. Less of the bitter, astringent and harsh tasting vegetables during Uttarayana, more of the sour, salty and sweet during Dakshinayana. The physical powers of Humans peak during the Hemanta and Sisira Ritus and touch their nadir during Greeshma and Vasanta. The health of the human body fluctuates with the season and the effects of climate.

As the climate progressively cools during Hemanta, the human body itself contracts externally. The pores and such outlets for energy and heat close, channeling internal energy to activity such as digestion, and increasing demand for nutrition. The body grows weak if deprived of nutrients. Sweets, sour and salty foods in large quantity can satisfy this demand and are suitable to these seasons. Nights are long and one may often awake feeling hungry, and it is appropriate to take a meal before the massage, to alleviate Vatadoshas. It is the season for vigorous exercise, followed by application of selected oils, which are later removed with green gram powder and a wash with clean water, before anointing and applying cosmetics. Typical foods are high in fat and meat content, and in sugar, milk, oils and black gram. Wines based on wheat may be drunk. Hot water should be used for washing, whether for hands and feet or bathing.

**Seasonal Conduct and Health**
Bedding is made from woollen rugs and material that retains heat. The body should be exposed to bright sunshine, but protective clothing such as shoes and gloves should be employed otherwise. Such procedure should be followed even more rigorously during Hemanta than Sisira as the cold intensifies. Couples can fulfill their sexual desires to capacity.

With the onset of Vasanta, the accumulated Kapha in the body liquefies and digestive powers wane. Emetics and nasal medication is indicated at the beginning of Vasanta Ritu itself, to drain the Kapha. Suitable nutrition is still required, along with some exercise and application of dry Udvartana, to remove some of the fat which has accumulated in the previous season. Drakshasava, a weak wine may be drunk, preferably diluted with honey, water or solutions of ginger. Protection offered by shady places may be required during the day, and exposure to sunlight, especially when from the East is to be avoided, although nights in the outdoors, bathed in moonlight, may be pleasant. Heavy, salty, sour foods or an abundance of sweets are certainly not recommended, while daytime sleeping is prohibited.

During Greeshma, the sun is often scorching and exercise should be light, preferably in the early hours. Pungent and sour buffalo-milk and cooled in the night air is a healthy drink for this season. Sleeping in the open air is recommended at night.

This season then gives way to the Varsha Ritu, as the monsoon hits with vapour laden winds and the rains set in. There is slush on the ground and humidity in the air and conditions are ripe for the vitiation of the tridoshas. Food must be such as to maintain their balance. Purgatives, enemas and emetics, food that is rich in fibre content, such as old, starchy grain or corn, that will clean the large intestine must be taken. Mudga, which is freely available during this period, is a good food as it is easily digested. Foods may contain some sour, salty and fat content. Panchakola and curds with medicated salts are excellent tonics. Wine may be drunk, but diluted with water. These should be imbibed warm.

Protection is required for the feet and hot water baths for the nights. Sleep during daytime is proscribed.

Sharad follows, with the sun often bright, exciting the accumulated Pitta of the Varsha season. Ghee, in which bitter herbs, such as *Tiktakaghrita* or *Mahatitakaghrita*, have been mixed, is a good antidote for such conditions. In days of yore, blood letting was often performed during this season. Purgatives which enhance the removal of Pitta may be useful. Diet may consist of *Patolas*, vegetables, sugar, meat, emblic myrobalans mixed into sweet, bitter and/or astringent tasting and easily digestible stuff. Hamsodaka, simply water which is left out in the sun and so, heats up during the day and cools at night, is a good tonic. To be avoided are overeating of any kind, and foods that contain fats, oils, curds, alcohol and alkaline substances. Day-time sleep is again proscribed, but people are normally healthy during this season.

As one Ritu merges into the next, so should the type of diet change gradually. Importance is ascribed to *Ritu Sandhi*, which is the name given to the period of transition between one season and the next. In lore, Ritu Sandhi is the period for extraordinarily unnatural conditions, evil planetary positions and curses of evil spirits and the anger of *Rakshashas* (demons) who poison the atmosphere and vitiate water. It is said to be a time of quarrels at home and disputes with members of family. The countryside is said to be vitiated when entire parts of it are changed, calamities occur, unusual smells pervade large tracts. Vegetation is affected by pestilence, victuals taste foul, pests of all kind proliferate and even animal behaviour changes and is at its most bestial.

Generally, it must be noted that the meals that are taken should harmonise with the season and certain flavours suit certain seasons.

# 8

# DOSHAS AND HEALTH

Each human body is nothing but a miniature version of the world, where Space arranges for the distribution of supplies as well as matter to different locations for the convenience of respective users. Fire symbolises energy processes, Water for drinking, growing of plants and as a translocuter, so do Kapha, Pitta and Vata for the body. Panchamahabhutas are present in every human being – *Akashabhuta* governs all the immaterial elements and functions, *Vayubhuta* the material, *Agnibhuta* the chemical and metabolic, and *Prithvibhuta* the anabolic, the additive and regenerative. These Bhutas are supplied or created from the food and medicine that the body imbibes.

Ayurveda places medicines in three broad categories. These are:

- *Balya* – the tonics and the nutrients
- *Deepanapachana* – stimulants for digestion and assimilation
- *Uttejaka* – repair agents for all other body parts

Doshas are ever-present in the body and generally coexist in harmony with each other, although they are very different in their properties. They are also used to existing in imbalanced states for long periods. For example, blood which is carried in the *Dhamani* (artery) is in a charged condition and gradually gets depleted (or vitiated) by the time it gets to the veins, and then to the heart for the process of charging to begin afresh.

Thus, it is natural for depleted or vitiated blood to be in the body and such blood does not produce any ill effects, subject to its normal cycle of re-purification in the lungs.

Similarly the intrinsic qualities of the Universe, the *Trigunas*, namely *Satva, Rajas* and *Tamas* are also ever-present in the body and work together. **Satvaguna**, like Vayu or space is incapable of being vitiated. **Rajoguna**, determinant of activity, can be likened to Pitta; while **Tamoguna**, determinant of stability and continuance, can be likened to Kapha.

## Normal States of Vata, Pitta and Kapha

There are five classes of Vata in the body and are called its *Pancha-vata*. The *Pranavayu* is centred in the head and pervades the heart, lung and neck. Acting in conjunction with the *Sadhaka Pitta, Vyanavayu* and the *Avalambaka Kapha,* it produces intellect, the subconcious mind and the heart and organs. The *Udanavayu* is centred in the lungs and heart and pervades the navel, neck and nose. Acting in conjunction with the *Vata Kapha, Vatapitta* and the *Bodhaka Kapha,* it produces voluntary actions, speech, skin colour and tone, strength, skills, enthusiasm and memory. *Vyanavayu* is centred in the heart, but can move through the entire body rapidly for motor functions, walking, expansion and contraction of muscles, the hand and feet, controlling the voice and all the physical functions of the body. It operates in conjunction with the Avalambaka Kapha as well as with four other Kaphas and five Pittas.

*Samanavayu,* centred in the small intestine, moves through the large, deglutinising and digesting food. It differentiates the *Sara* (nutrient) from the *Kitta* (excreta), operating together with *Kledaka Kapha* and *Alochaka Kapha.*

*Apnavayu,* centred in the lower abdomen, moves through the large intestine, the head, thighs and the generative organs, dispelling excreta of all kind, faeces, semen, urine, foetus and menses. It operates together with *Bhrajaka Pitta* and *Kledaka Kapha*.

There are five types of Pitta in the body. *Pachaka Pitta* is present in the small intestine and it assists in the digestion of food and formation of refuse, operating together with Samanavayu, Vyanavayu and Kledaka Kapha. It also helps synergise the other four Pittas. *Ranjaka Pitta*, in the stomach, assists with chyme (*Rasa*), together with Vyanavayu and Kledaka Kapha. *Alchaka Pitta*, in the eyes helps in the normal functioning of vision in conjunction with Vyanavayu, Pranavayu and Kledaka Kapha. *Bhrajaka Pitta*, in the skin helps in maintaining normal skin tone in conjunction with Vyanavayu, Kledaka Kapha and all tissues in the body.

Five Kaphas are present in the body. *Avalambaka Kapha* is centred in the stomach and produces chyme and digestive fluids in conjunction with Samanyavayu, Pachakapitta and Vyanavayu.

*Bodhaka Kapha* is present in the tongue and provides taste discrimination, acting in conjunction with Udanavayu and Pranavayu. *Tarpaka Kapha* is present in the head and nourishes all the organs in conjunction with Vyanavayu and Pranavayu. *Shleshmaka Kapha* is present in the joints to transport the vatas to their respective places of function, while simultaneously assisting them.

Eighty distinct diseases are linked with the vitiation of Vata, forty with the vitiation of Pitta and twenty with that of Kapha. Charaka described the doshas in their non-vitiated condition and their effect on the body. Doshas are called the *Dhatus* of life as they shape the body, are vital to existence and balanced properly help the body live long and healthily. While Vata is concentrated in the lower part of the body, Pitta is concentrated in the centre, and Kapha at the top. All three must exist for life to be. Blood may be conceptualised as a mixture of the three doshas or as a fourth dosha in itself, as it

36

is critical for life. The doshas themselves are regulated by the Atma and in spite of dietary and situational changes, these are kept balanced. Quality nutrition, however, is a requisite for them to be so regulated and provides health, happiness and longevity.

The food that is ingested produces Rasa in the stomach, which goes on through the bloodstream to produce blood, flesh, whether muscle, tissue or fat, bones and marrow, Sukra, Ojas and glandular secretions, the constituents of the five sensory organs, tendons and cartilage. A byproduct of food is *kitta*, or *mala*, or excreta, which leaves the body as faeces, urine, sweat or as Vata, Pitta and Kapha, excretions out of the body through orifices and cavities, the mouth, nose, eyes and ears, even the minute roots of hair. Disease can be due to ingestion of uncompatible food. While some excreta may be retained in the body to an extent without causing disease, the retention of excreta produced in the cavities of the body, such as urine must be immediately expelled to avoid disease.

The taste of the food hints at the type of dhatu it will provide and so the dosha that it will help generate. Rasa is the first product of digestion, Kapha Dhatu through sweets, Pitta through the sour victuals in the middle of the meal and Vata through the pungent foods at the end as the digested food enters the large intestine and the fluid part dries up.

In their fresh, charged form, while they are useful in their functions and before they get vitiated, they are called dhatus. Vata will produce and regulate respiration and all the organs of the body down to the cellular and molecular and atomic levels. It will maintain digestion and the assimilation processes. Pitta will also aid digestion, produce thirst and hunger, maintain vision and those body parts which are soft, a healthy appearance of the skin and contribute to the compassion memory, happiness, preferences, bravery and intelligence. Kapha will provide with the physical aspects –

body weight and structure, strength, fortitude, generosity and forgiveness, endurance and lack of greed. Vata distributes the Rasa which is produced to all parts of the body for basic energy. If Rasa is not properly formed, it will obstruct the *Srotas* or channels of the body, causing disease. Vata also distributes Pitta and Kapha. Qualities associated with Vata are coldness, lightness, roughness, harshness, subtleness, excessiveness and motility. Qualities associated with Pitta are lightness, foulness, heat, oiliness, speed, and glandular secretions; those associated with Kapha are coldness, heaviness, motionlessness, sweetness and oiliness.

Treatment of disorders consists of supplementing one dosha with the other. For example, the heaviness of Kapha with the lightness of Pitta; the heat of Pitta by the coldness of Vata; the motionlessness of Kapha by the motivity of Vata, or by the speed of Pitta; the softness of Kapha by the hardness of Pitta. Treatment of improper formation of Rasa, which leads to a condition called Ama (undigested food particles) and the underlying cause for a number of ailments can be treated with fasting or light diet, digestive stimulants, and in advanced cases, with *Panchakarma* therapy.

# 9

# SPIRITUAL AND MENTAL HEALTH

From earlier ages, the role of public swasthavritta or the issue of public health has played a role per the prevailing demands of the public. Due to either negligence or sheer misconduct, the public would be afflicted with some disease or contagion, or the other suffered. The sages, it is said, took pity on them and started the Science of Ayurveda.

It was the sage, Athreya, who initiated the collection of medicine and medical treatment of the public, suffering from a number of complications. The authorities on Ayurveda, then declared that their main purpose was to provide relief to the public, those in real distress and that this was their religious duty. Treatment was of two types:

- **Daivavyapasraya** – methods of treating disease through propitiation and employment of supernatural powers.

- **Sattavavajaya** – methods of treating disease through mental control.

*Daivavyapasraya* consists of treating disease with *Mantras* (recitation and invocation to the Almighty and super-beings), use of special stones with beneficial and medicinal properties, worship and determination of the auspicious, through offerings and fire services, through sacrifice to super-beings, observing vows and fasts, and prostrating oneself as many times as required, before the deities. Ayurveda was considered to be a branch of *Atharvaveda*, employing *Yajnachakra*, the cycle of exchange of assets from a human being to The Superior One, as well as to inferiors.

*Sattavavajaya* is based on the concept that the mind can control the body and a majority of ailments arise from unhealthy occupation and the presence of worry. It recognises that a host of unhealthy conditions, including worldwide disturbances can cause aberrations in mental environment.

Mental health plays an important role not only at the level of individuals, but also on public health. Conditions, such as epilepsy, mania, insanity, all stem from the mind. It is said that the peaceful condition of mind was lost by Lord Shiva and this caused the expulsion of major chunks of population, leading to unhealthy living conditions and so adversely affecting public health. Traces of this can be found in the Ramayana, when public tranquility was disturbed when Ram was banished, and then again, when Sita was degraded from her queenhood. That period of the epoch was immediately followed by a period of calamity and contagion.

Charaka has aptly described the importance of maintaining one's own mental balance, for every human being. Loss of balance is known to be widespread in every calamity, such as in time of plague and other epidemic outbreaks. In the Bhagavad Geeta, public equanimity is termed as Lokasamagraha – a divine song sung by Lord Sri Krishna to set right the disturbed mental health of Arjuna.

# 10

# SATVADI GUNAS AND HEALTH

Ayurveda is of the opinion that the mind itself is capable of becoming vitiated due to the vitiation of the *Gunas* that make up the mind. When this happens, mental disease is the inevitable result, just as vitiation of the Doshas cause physiological disease.

*Prakriti*, or nature itself, is said to be made up of the three Gunas, or qualities. These are called *Satvaguna, Rajoguna* and *Tamoguna* respectively. The first of these, namely Satva, cannot be vitiated and abundance of the same will promote mental equilibrium and health. A Satvic constitution is therefore a naturally healthy one. Tamoguna and Rajoguna, however, can be vitiated, and when this happens, the individual is prone to mental affliction. Because of the linkage of the mind to the body, mental health or lack of it is a percussor to the physical condition. The importance of Satvaguna, as a necessity for mental health, is highlighted in the Bhagavad Geeta. Both the Geeta and Charaka, advocate Yoga, which may be of many sorts, for attaining Moksha. But, in order to practise Yoga, one has to have a healthy body in the first place and a healthy body is only possible with a healthy mind. Satvaguna, encompasses Truth, the power of acquisition of knowledge, peace of mind and all such qualities. Rajoguna is the quality that produces feelings of likes and dislikes, biases, distress, dissatisfaction and such. Tamas is the quality that is instinctive, the id, if you like, that is animal response, the libido and the objectionable. According to tenets of Patanjali Yoga, these three naturally occurring qualities in nature, or Prakriti, are present in the human body as Doshas. The Bhagavad Geeta goes on to state that a healthy body itself promotes Satvaguna, and coupled with the realisation of external truth, this may dispel death, even at an advanced age.

The diseases of the body and the mind are thus, interrelated and interdependent.

Qualities that may be called Satvic include – loyalty, humanity (humaneness), gratitude, honour, valour, pride, thirst for knowledge, fairness, faith, belief in God, -intelligence, memory, charity, enterprise.

Qualities that may be categorised as being of the Rajoguna kind, include – anger, breakdowns, hatred, greed, envy, revenge, mischief, arrogance, grief.

Qualities that fall into the Tamoguna kind, include – pessimism, dejection, cynicism, stupidity, ignorance, promiscuity, slothfulness, laziness, prone to influences, specially the harmful, lack of control over actions and inability to apply judgement.

With the acquisition of Satvaguna, one can gain knowledge of the sciences – Jnana and Vijnana, self-control, fearlessness, detachment and the judgement to value the materialistic and the frivolous, as they are. The Satvic practises *Dhriti* (steadfastness), *Smriti* and *Buddhi,* and with each such practise, raises his Satvic levels further, while controlling Tamas and Rajo. The highly Satvic are capable of exhibitions of paranormal powers, the ability to disappear, of foretelling, teleporting and remembering past lives. This state is known as *Vasitva,* and the pure or ultimate Satvic is one who is completely free of either joy or sorrow.

# 11

# MENTAL HEALTH

Ayurveda postulates that mental health is of supreme importance for healthy living, and in order to live happily, the mind and body must both be in balanced condition.

**The Nature of the Mind** – the mind is the centre that is responsible for controlling every facet of physical activity of its owner. External actions and stimuli can govern the mind. Favourable treatment from others results in feelings of happiness. Unhappiness results when this is not so. Thus, it appears that to be able to command or demand favourable response from one's environment, be it nature or other beings, is a dire neccessity.

Per the tenets of Ayurveda, however, the surest way to rule or influence others is to control and regulate one's own self. This is an *Avyakta* (unmanifested) principle. That there is an *Atma* (soul) which is self-existing, endless, indestructible and unmanifested, is also an Avyakta, from which is born *Buddhi* (intelligence), which in turn leads to the sense of self or *Ahamkar,* Aham being self. From this is born the existence of Akash and the very particles of matter, organs of subuniversal bodies. All that is manifested is derived from the unmanifested and this, the manifested, is divided between what may be understood by mankind and what is beyond his understanding. Some of the unseen and unfelt may be understood by inference.

## Prakriti

Prakriti, or Nature, is said to be composed of the five Bhutas, as well as Avyakta, Buddhi and Ahamkara. Ergo, it follows that every individual must have these eight as constituents of his or her system. In fact, these, along with the fifteen organs, constitute the make up of every human. These fifteen organs are called the *Vikaras* of Prakriti – manifestations of the cosmic phenomena. Five which are intelligence or Buddhi based, five sensory organs and five motor organs. The Vikaras, being manifestations, are mutable, and accordingly, the mind, which is a Vikara, may be moulded as one likes, or even change when influenced. Under such influence, the mind can transform itself to any one of the *Shuddha* (Satvic or pure), Rajasa or Tamasa types. In living beings, the Avyakta becomes its soul and remains unmutable. The Shuddha mind is the normal or healthy and pure mind, but the other two states are considered to be vitiated states of mind. Rajasa minds are those which are overly passionate, obsessive or inflamed; while Tamasa minds are those lacking in the sensibilities.

Behaviour patterns of the Shuddha mind and body will reflect in its actions, exhibiting qualities and traits that may be called noble. Such as straightforwardness, compassion, generosity, gratitude, fortitude, intelligence, initiative, ability to memorise, faith, comprehension, forbearance, tolerance, and a sense of perspective and some detachment from worldly affairs.

The Rajasa mind and body will reflect the negative traits of discontentment, unhappiness, covetousness, egotism, deceit, cruelty, hypocrisy, conceit, anger and frivolity.

The Tamasa mind and body will reflect the negative traits of ignorance and the inability to judge the subjective from the objective, dullness, lethargy, misbehaviour, an aversion to the religious and enlightening, and a lack of character, devotion and pity. Should such a mind not be well-guided, the organs will be in a state of excitation and the body prone to disease, often of the life-threatening kind.

The practise of Yoga, which teaches both discipline and direction, helps the mind to function properly, thus bestowing not only normality, but also powers that can be considered extraordinary and even super-human. Disease is inevitable with loss of balance of mind because such loss results in the vitiation of the Doshas.

### Achieving a Shuddha Mind Condition

Ayurveda believes that the way we behave governs our mould of mind. Thus, by consciously practising the 'noble' we will be able to enjoy a Shuddha mind state, which in turn will contribute to the well-being of the body.

Being truthful always, controlling one's temper under all circumstances, avoiding any kind of addiction, specially for wine and women, avoiding hurting, maiming and killing, keeping the mind filled with pure thoughts, curbing passion, being patient with others, doing good to others, and so on, are all prerequisites for achieving the desired condition of mind. Recognition of mentors, whether they be religious people, men of learning or simply the old and the wise, for the guidance that they are able to provide, all goes a long way in building a behaviour pattern such as listed above.

Factors that lead to breakdowns in correct behaviour must be avoided. These include, irregularity in the daily duties, and improper intake of food – whether too much or of the wrong kind. One needs to concentrate on one's behaviour, often requiring a very conscious effort on our part. Being gentlemanly, when in a difficult situation. Or else, steering away from a course of action. Often, the first step to such a practise is to begin with the home, with relatives and friends, before extending such norms vis-à-vis the public. Effort is also required in controlling the organs of one's physical body, by trying and improving one's knowledge, by analysing and reflecting on routine and day to day activity, as well as on actions for the future. In the words of the sages – He who controls his senses and behaves as a gentleman, will have a heart as clear as the cleanest of mirrors and his mind will shine, as calm and tranquil as an oil lamp which gives light in the service of others.

# MEASURES TO MAINTAIN HEALTH

Measuring the state of health of any being employs routes which may be either direct or indirect. The direct route is the one where measurement or examination of indicators determine whether one is healthy or unhealthy. The indirect route is the one where one arrives at the conclusion through inference.

To prevent disease by following the direct route, one requires sufficient information about what a healthy body is, what are disease-promoting conditions, about the disease and how it affects the body, measures for precautions, prevention, prophylaxis and treatment, and finally, preparing the mind by training it to fight off the disease. All this under what are often unusual and difficult circumstances.

To do so requires not only a concerted effort on the individual's part but also often drawing upon the services of dependable and selfless experts, when in need. To be said to be healthy, a person must be able to obstruct the spread of diseases, prevent their entering into the body, and dispel diseases if they happen to gain entry. When one is able to do these, he becomes self-confident about being able to maintain his own health.

**Understanding the activity of the body** – A body that is free from disease since birth, is thoroughly capable of maintaining its condition of health, subject to being provided proper nutrition. Nutrition provided must be agreeable to the body and must never produce uneasiness in either the body or the mind. So, although a particular food may be rich in nutrients and be easily digestible, it may still be unsuitable if it conjures squeamishness in the mind.

Actions and attitudes, usually such that are impulsive, and that provoke stress, are to be avoided.

**Effort is necessary to overcome disease** – Once afflicted by disease, one should realise that it is due to any among a range of conditions, such as idleness, lack of attention, impositions brought about by occupational activity and of own creation. The term for these is *Prajnaparadha*. By making a conscious effort at self-discipline, replenishment and treatment, one can be cured of the affliction.

**Physical urges** – Involuntary physical urges, such as sneezing, yawning, vomiting, shedding tears, clearing the bowels or passing urine, must never be stifled

**General** – Procrastination, insulting others, abusing one's body, whether to rigours of substance or travel, exposure to pathogen and adverse conditions, and the company we keep are all factors that take their toll on our health and promote the onset of disease.

**Role of recreation** – Appropriate recreation in small doses is certainly beneficial for health. Care must be exercised in ensuring, however, that recreational activity does not expose one to injury and exhaustion, contagion. Recreation, at the expense of the regimen of duties that one is expected to follow, is also harmful. Recreation that may lead to addiction, such as with narcotics and alcohol or tobacco is proscribed.

Sometimes, even harmless recreational activity can lead to endangered states of mind – a conversation can end up in argument and taunts, vituperation and condemnation. Such must be avoided.

Not all diseases are either avoidable or preventable. Accidents are known to happen, and accidental injury and disease can occur too. Quite often, though, these are curable, usually with outside help. Most human afflictions, however, are avoidable and preventable and may be cured with the application of a little effort on one's own part. Emaciation, for instance, may respond to simply providing a change in diet, adequacy of nutrient coupled with gentle exercise. Walking in the morning and evening, properly covered against inclement weather. On the other hand, if the condition persists, one may require advanced forms of treatment, such as **Panchakarma** treatment.

One must be prepared to fight the uncommon circumstances that life has a tendency to bring about during its course.

Successful treatment for what afflicts one, depends upon one's own appreciation of universal medical truths about creating a situation of health. The homily about a happy person being a healthy person is true. Imbalances in the body's make-up lead to sickness. Both body and mind are the storehouse for all manner stress, leading to unhappiness and so to sickness. Simple ignorance can lead to sickness. Overcome these and better health ensues.

Man can draw upon three modes of treatment for a cure. There are the superhuman measures – prayer, invocation and meditation. There is his own control over his functions and activity, and finally, all that is available in the corporeal world for treatment, such as equipment, procedures and medicine. This last encompasses the gamut available for exploration of the condition to its treatment; from the simple – an enema, applying ice or a hot water bag, taking temperature by thermometer, to the complex – EEGs and ECGs, scanning by ultrasound and MRI, and such. Modern systems are quite suitable for use along with Ayurveda. In combination, the two are synergistic.

The advice contained in the Ayurvedic texts are ageless, and basic as they are, are certain to allow their adherents a life of minimal ailment and contribute to both happiness and longevity in the process.

# 13

# THE DEFECTIVE CONSTITUTION

A defective constitution will cause a permanent state of unhealthiness in an individual. The constitution may be deemed defective owing to both mental and bodily (physical) causes. The physical abnormalities may be corrected with artificial limbs to make up for deformity or the sheer lack of limb, or by administering stimulant medicine. Mental abnormality with psychiatric care and schooling. However, a basically defective constitution is a storehouse for disease, per the tenets of Ayurveda, which has reserved terms such as *Vataja*, *Pittaja* and *Sleshmeja Prakritis* for such constitutions. The terminology determines the type of treatment required to alleviate the sickness stemming from the defect. Also, according to Ayurveda, there are three categories of sick people – those with predisposition of becoming indisposed, the pitiable and the punishable.

**The Easily Indisposed** – People in this group are prone to illness. Their *Tridoshas* are not in a natural state of equilibrium and they may be of the *Doshika*, the *Samsargika* or the *Sannipatika* types, permanently indisposed constitutions, which respond to treatment and need not, therefore, be permanently ill.

**The Pitiable** – To illustrate by giving examples – dwarfs, giants, albinos, people born with physical deformities, those who are constitutionally over or underweight, all qualify for

51

inclusion in this group. Even though their physical bodies may not conform to normality, they may be generally healthy in that they do not suffer from illness. In some cases, the condition can be corrected to an extent or may not even require any. While both being abnormally underweight and overweight are defects, in Ayurveda, being underweight is preferred to being overweight and in cases not deemed worthy of further treatment.

**The Punishable** – Born healthy, those in this group fall prey to disease because of personal habit. Examples of this group can include people such as policemen, guards, watchmen and menials, who, by accepting such occupation, have allowed themselves to jeopardise their health. This group also includes students appearing for competitive examinations, research scholars, doctors, advocates and businessmen who sacrifice their own health in the interest of others. The worst in this category are those who put themselves at risk for addiction and pleasure, such as those who visit prostitutes, and criminals risking prison sentences.

# 14

# OJAS AND HEALTH

**Ojas** is the term given by Charaka to the purest kind of Dhatu or material in the body. Vagbhata and Sushrutha have all contributed to the concept of Ojas as an invisible source of strength and energy in the body and its role in the well being of the body being secondary only to the presence of the soul. It was postulated by Sushrutha, that Shukra (semen) is a form of Ojas, but other forms are the **Sleshmas**, reddish-yellow when in blood, white in its pure Sleshma form. It is attributed with the power of soothing and pacifying the body, providing energy, freshness, brightness and the very life-force. Loss of Ojas, it is postulated, results in grief and dejection, loss of the peace of mind and mental control. It is created out of the food that one eats, the same as all the other dhatus, the heat and the energy in the body.

It is measured by the effects that it produces in the body. It is formed in an individual from the time that a foetus starts forming and pervades all over the body, being carried by the Pranavayu of the Vatadosha. Sruti believed that the Ojas is the *Prana* (life-force) itself. Swami Vivekananda, in rather more modern times, has said that it is *Pranashakti* indeed, in his book on Rajayoga. Ayurveda thought has it that it is vital for strength, both physical and mental, and should be preserved by all human beings. It is the essence of all body constituents or Dhatus starting from Rasa to Rakta to Shukra although it changes to Mala for excretion, when vitiated, and in this state performs no useful function.

Food aids in muscular growth, promote the formation of Ojas in the body, and once formed this can be stored by the body for use when required. Symptoms of plentiful Ojas are the signs of glowing health, pleasantness of temperament, normal functioning of all organs, a strong, well-formed body and good skin and appearance.

Food of the type that generates Rajas and Tamas Gunas in the body will vitiate and deplete the amount of Ojas in any body. Satvic foods, on the other hand, increase the amount of Ojas. Symptoms of its depression are – loss of taste for food, fear of even minor things, loss of skin tone, heaviness, swelling and inflammation, lethargy, difficulty in movement, loss of strength. In its ultimate stages, loss of Ojas leads to emaciation and death.

# 15

# PERSPECTIVES ABOUT FOOD

To state the obvious, food and water are essential for life. Food is the sustainer of life, whereas, water is its reviver. This is universal for the growth and development of all living beings, including humans. Among the human race, however, the sources of the food that we eat, the type of food that we eat, and its very cooking may be at great variance from culture to culture, from location to location. These can vary greatly among even neighbouring families.

Ayurveda accords food its due importance. It has classified food depending on source of origin, content and characteristics, and effects on the human body. It has also studied the fact that not only what, but also the way we eat, affects the way we feel and our health.

Broadly, food may be classified as derived from one of three sources – animal, vegetable or mineral. Whatever the source or combination of sources, that food the we eat must be *Panchbhautic.* That is, it must provide us with a suitable intake of and replenishment for the five Bhutas that constitute our material selves.

The very taste of food is an indicator of the bhutas that it is capable of replenishing, and each individual taste, such as sweetness for example, is made of the combination of two bhutas being predominant in that particular food.

The six, individual taste types are linked to the Panchamahabhutas as listed under –

1. Sweet        : Prithvibhuta  + Apbhuta
2. Sour         : Agnibhuta     + Prithvibhuta
3. Salty        : Agnibhuta     + Apbhuta
4. Bitter       : Akashabhuta   + Vayubhuta
5. Pungent      : Agnibhuta     + Vayubhuta
6. Astringent   : Prithvibhuta  + Vayubhuta

The vegetable kingdom provides all these taste types, except the salty, which comes from a mineral source and is abundantly available in the oceans and the seas. Fruits predominate in providing the sweet, sour and pungent.

Water is a form of Apbhuta, while air is a form of Vayubhuta, and the human body, generally, has an affinity for what is sweet.

Eating food of a variety of taste, therfore, results in imbibing the many bhutas, thereby automatically providing for a balanced intake. Foods also differ in their *Veerya* (potency) and this has led to certain conventions of Ayurvedic practise, in the taste of food and medication, and even in terms of the drugs administered to alleviate a condition. For example, the sweet to follow the pungent, or to counterbalance the sour and salty; the bitter and astringent to counterbalance the salty, the sour to balance the pungent and also the bitter and astringent. The pungent has attributes which are the opposite of the bitter and astringent. Generally, the bitter and the astringent are used in conjunction. This is not for the medicinal or nutritional functions, but merely as a matter of taste.

### Prescriptions For the Way We Eat

From the times of Charaka and earlier, the way food is eaten has been deemed to be of importance. Charaka advised – take food when it is hot, and with a sufficient quantity of ghee, in a pleasant place, chewing the food properly and ingesting neither too quickly nor too slowly. One should not talk or laugh or weep during mealtime.

Vagbhata advises the would-be eater to bathe or wash before eating. As the first step, an offering should be made to God, and then to cattle and children.

When and how much we eat are very important in Ayurveda and 'proper' is the operative word for both. Fruits should be eaten at the start of the meal, and sour and salty foods towards the conclusion, as sweet and fatty foods are not quickly digested. Intake should be such that, a third of the stomach is filled with solids and a third with liquids, leaving a third of the stomach for the production of the tridoshas, Vata, Pitta and Kapha. Food should be eaten fresh and hot, and one should not eat less than the quantities outlined above as the empty capacity will be prone to flatulence and belching can result.

Constipation and loose motions (*Udvartana*) shorten life.

When eating, focus on the meal – excitement, emotions and outbursts of any sort are proscribed during mealtimes. The mind is to be kept free of sorrow, shame and feeling of dejection.

Overeating causes indigestion and aggravates Vata, Pitta and Kapha, The symptoms of vitiation of Vata can be – shooting pain, bleeding from the nose, body pain, pain in the waist and the back, dry mouth, contraction of the blood vessels, fainting and delirium. Symptoms of provocation of Pitta may include fever, burning sensation in the body, thirst, unconsciousness and delirium, and aggravation of Kapha may produce vomiting, loss of taste for food, delay in digestion, fever with rigour, disinterestedness and heaviness in the body.

Treatment for being overweight is corrected by administering medicines which alleviate the Vata and Kapha Doshas, by prescribing a regimen of exercise, of mental stimulation, of application. Treatment for the underweight may be just dietary in nature, with some treatment for the behaviour problems that such a person may be associated with, such as irritability or anger, which may require a soothing type of regimen or drugs termed as *Jeevaneeya,* served in concoctions derived from milk, curd, ghee, wheat and barley. Regimen may consist of enhanced sleep periods such as daytime sleeping, improving sleeping comforts, such as a softer bed and shielding from excitement and anxiety. Foods may include larger intake of rice and pulses and wine. Dress often helps this condition. Clean garments certainly help and so does the colour white.

Medicine administered for weight conditions can be of either the *Rasayana* or *Vajikarna* type. Ayurveda believes that meat and dairy products are principal contributors to an overweight condition, and that practise of Abhyanga will help in gaining weight. But whatever the weight condition, diet and nutrition are essentials for basic functioning.

# SWASTHAVRITTA IN WOMEN

The male and female human bodies are similar in almost all characteristics, including the Doshas and almost all the Dhatus, although there are some differences owing to the role that the female of the species plays for procreation. Women have the ability of becoming pregnant and bearing children, whereas men cannot. Constitutionally, the Dhatus in the female and the male are entirely similar, except that the Shukra in the male is replaced by the *Arthava* in the female. Structurally, while the feet, the hands, the head, hair, trunk and most internal organs have a commonality for both the sexes, females differ from males in having a vulva and two breasts. The Malas and seven Ashayas are common to both sexes, but women have an extra Ashaya, the *Garbhashaya*.

At between twelve and sixteen years of age in India, girls starts menstruating. This is a period of great sensitivity from the health point of view and Ayurveda stresses that great attention be paid to avoiding exposure, as such exposures may result in long term illness and ill-health. Based upon the practises of that time, some of the recommendations of Ayurveda proscribed sleeping by day, avoiding having to shed tears, and not applying eye salve and cosmetics. Massage in oil was also proscribed during this period, as well as any action which might provoke excessive emotion and physical exertion. Depending upon its level, even what appears to be harmless activity, such as running, laughing, storytelling and exposure to the external environment such as loud sounds or the weather, require to be moderated.

The appearance of the menses signals that the woman is ready to conceive in order to maintain the continuity of the race and during the period of her menstruation, it is strictly prohibited for her to be involved in the sexual act, as this may lead to diseases. During pregnancy, she has to nourish her foetus through her body fluids in addition to nourishing her own body and so, her Swasthavritta differs from that of a man. She requires special treatment to supplement for the extra requirement. Prescriptions for the pregnant woman were laid down by both Sushrutha and Vagbhata and consist of a list of "do's" and "dont's". The "dont's" include excessive indulgence in sex, lifting heavy weights, sitting in one place for a long period of time, sleeping on her back, overeating, imbibing alcohol, eating meat and withholding the calls of nature. The dont's also include not getting into provoking circumstances that affect the mind, such as situations that build fear, lamentation, anger, vertigo. Wearing garments which are red in colour is also proscribed, as is taking any kind of emetic or purgative for the first eight months of pregnancy.

The "dos" include gentle indulgency in her cravings and wants as these are believed to be linked with the foetus. Her longings are to be provided for and a diet with plentiful milk, butter and ghee is good for her. It is recognised that owing to complications which may arise from her condition, medication may be required, but this has to be kept to as mild as possible. By now, the foetus is fully developed and its body parts have formed. One complication which is anticipated is itching, that appears in the seventh month of pregnancy in different parts of her body, coupled, possibly, with hot flushes in her hands and feet, while she develops folds of skin on her abdomen, chest and stomach. This is to be treated with plentiful water intake and a diet rich in fruit which is light and easy to digest

– sweet berries and the pulp of sweet fruits. Salt and fat intake should both be reduced and the skin folds which have appeared should be massaged with sandalwood oil.

The role of Ojas is particularly important in the eighth month of pregnancy as the foetus constantly changes its position. Deprived of Ojas, the woman will be unhappy, but milk or ghee with boiled rice prove good sources for such replenishment. Meanwhile, she should be given *Uttaravasti*, composed of a sweet-based unguent through her vulva, to maintain its softness and elasticity. Administration of enemas are recommended to clear the large intestine properly. This enema consists of *Shatahva* oil, ghee and rock salt along with a decoction of *Milaka* and sweet berries.

During her ninth month of pregnancy, her diet should consist of solid food, for example, rice and ghee with meat gruel. Uttaravasti continues, and in addition, a cotton swab soaked in water containing juices extracted from the Vata-alleviating leaves of medicinal plants, should be kept in her vulva.

Even after she delivers her child, her special regime of Swasthavritta should continue. She may be prone to pain, the common locations being the head and the stomach. Some remedies for this are – a mixture of ghee and Yavakshara, or, a decoction of coriander seeds flavoured with jaggery, pepper, cardamom, long pepper, *Tamala* leaf and cinnamon.

For the first two to three days after delivery, when hungry, she should be given a drink of ghee and *Panchakola*. Panchakola is a combination of long pepper, *Pippalimola*, *Cavaka*, *Chitraka* and ginger. For slaking her thirst, water sweetened with jaggery and containing extracts of Vata subduing drugs, should be provided. When these have been given, her abdomen should be rubbed with ghee or oil and bound and wrapped with a piece of cloth. Once the medicinal ghee has been digested, the woman should be bathed and this is to be followed with the Panchakola gruel. For the first fifteen days after delivery, she may also be given a decoction of an ounce of black *Jeera* on a daily basis.

After the first three days have elapsed and till the seventh day, she should be given gruel from the boiled pulp of *Vidari* drugs, mixed with either ghee or milk. Fattening foods are good for her at this point. Having just been through the trauma of labour and childbirth and the related stresses of growth of foetus, loss of body fluids and the press of the growing body on her internal body parts, she is in weakened condition and susceptible to diseases. Disease at this stage will seriously threaten her well being; much more than normally, since she is at her least resilient. Two tonics will help – an ounce of *Dashamularista,* twice a day with water, and five grams of *Soubhagya Shunti Rasayana,* twice a day.

Thereafter, she reverts to her normal, common and proper regime of Swasthavritta. Around her fiftieth year, her menses will stop and she will no longer function as a childbearer. From this point on, her Swasthavritta will be similar to any man's, though it may be noted that men can continue to father children beyond fifty.

# 17

# SWASTHAVRITTA IN
# THE YOUNG AND THE OLD

Broadly, children may be categorised into three classes as under:

1. Those dependant purely on milk for sustenance
2. Those drawing sustenance on a combination of milk and food
3. Those dependant purely on food for sustenance

The first category of children, that is, those dependent purely on milk for sustenance, are the least prone to, disease, as long as they get their milk from their mother or a wet nurse, or even a substitute source which is free from infection. When a mother, who is herself malnourished or of irregular habits, is the source of the milk, the child is unlikely to contract disease, but the possibility of infection increases when a wet nurse or a substitute is the source of milk. *Mother's milk is the ideal and best food for an infant and there is no substitute for it.* It is sterile in the sense of being free from infection and entirely requisite in its composition of proteins, fats and carbohydrates necessary for the growth of the child. Insufficient supply of mother's milk creates a problem and might require treatment for the child.

Once weaned, the child is exposed to, and thus, susceptible to disease. It is these second and third categories of children who should follow the regime of Swasthavritta. The regime is similar to the one advocated for men in general, except for the exclusion of Vyayama (exercise), Tambula Sevana (chewing betel leaves) and Dhumrapana (medicated smoking). The child, while growing continuously, will develop from a demanding being (dependant on others for the fulfillment of its wants) to a being interested in an environment outside of itself and gradual independence and self-sufficiency.

The aged are characterised with loss of vitality and infirmity, and an increase in dependancy on others for fulfilling their needs. They will lose interest in the environment and exhibit a process of withdrawal into themselves. The more such signs they show, the poorer their health conditions, and they will require the services of such as, homes for the aged, whether State or Central Government or voluntary agencies.

# 18

# THE RIGHT CONDUCT
# (SADVRITTA)

The way we behave and go about conducting ourselves has a bearing on the condition of our health. Improper conduct and the lack of a code of etiquette, whether with our own selves, either body or mind, or with others, is detrimental to our health. A basic truth, it is worth examining Charaka's postulates on what constitutes proper conduct. His tenets – One should never lie, nor, covet another's property. One should not provoke enmity, nor find faults with others and disrespect confidentiality.

In keeping with his times, he declared that one should – not ride untamed animals, never vomit without covering the mouth, never blow one's nose or pick one's teeth in front of others. One should not go against one's superiors and not mix with one's inferiors. To avoid beasts and serpents, fire and water.

Food is to be taken after a bath, with a jewel in at least one finger and free of dust. Food must be taken after checking that the location is a suitable one, and that it is sacrilegious to eat, spit or excrete when engaged in offering prayer or sacrifice to God. One is not to remain in a state of anger or hysterical joy for any length of time – control is intrinsic to the proper code of conduct. One should practise the spirit of celibacy, indulging in sex on occasion, abstaining from such pleasure-seeking outside one's home.

**General Rules of Conduct for the Male:** Not to engage in sexual intercourse when his spouse in menstruating, ill, otherwise physically incapacitated or such, indecent in appearance, behaving badly, unwilling, preoccupied or not in the proper mental frame. Sexual acts are not be conducted while sleeping in the vicinity of a peepul tree, at the crossroads, in the garden, at the crematorium, water house or at the chemists and in the temple. Such acts are not to be conducted when the spouse is in the midst of her household duties or when there are guests at home, when fasting, being medically treated or about to answer the call of nature. Cohabitation should be in a discreet and suitable place. Adultery and incest are taboo.

**General Rules of Conduct for the Female:** All the general rules for males that apply to cohabitation are also applicable for the female. Further, in case she is pregnant, she should avoid sleeping in the daytime, restrict the use of cosmetics such as kaajal to the eyes and any exposure that may have a detrimental effect on her foetus. She should consider the interests of her children and the effect that her actions may have on her family. Frivolous actions during pregnancy could affect the foetus drastically. It was believed that, frequent weeping resulted in a baby with defective eyesight, applying kaajal in blindness, oil baths in skin disease, hysteria in defective teeth, telling tall tales in talkativeness and if the mother-to-be was subjected to loud sounds, her baby would be born deaf. And that exposure to the wind and too much exercise for the mother would result in a child with an unmanageable nature.

A lady was to use a grass bed for sleeping and an earthen plate or a leaf for eating. For the first three days of her menses, she was supposed to fast, and then, the fast was to be broken only after an offering or sacrifice to God. For begetting a son, coitus was recommended for the fourth day after menses, after a bath. Coitus being reserved for alternate nights from this fourth to the twelfth night, if she really desired a son. Coitus on the other nights during this period would lead to begetting a daughter. So, for a son, the nights are the fourth, sixth, eighth, tenth and twelfth, and for a daughter the designated nights are the fifth, seventh, ninth and eleventh.

# 19

# THE IMPACT OF OCCUPATION ON HEALTH

That occupational activity is important to man but has its side effects is intrinsic to Ayurveda. *Vihara* is the term for such activity, and is performed when a person attains *Arthapurushartha*, *Purushartha* being the term for coming of age. There are three ways a person 'comes of age' – with *Dharmapurushartha* (spiritually), with *Karmapurushartha* (developing the ability of discharging duties and obligations) and with Arthapurushartha (developing the ability to generate material wealth and satisfy one's own needs). Occupation is important because it gives one the things he/she needs. It is the activity through which one contributes to the outside world, and also draws upon one's own collective requirements.

The main occupations during the times of Charaka were agriculture, government service, commerce, animal husbandry and public service. Referring to these, he propounded that the man who is not in a position to earn for his worldly requirements is the most sinful of all.

But occupation imposes pressures, both mental and physical and these leave their impact on the Doshas, thereby affecting health. Occupation also exposes one to the possibility of contagion and infection, which also affect health. Prevention and treatment of such diseases may be termed as Occupational Hygiene. To cope with the hardships of this worldly life, all that is required is to possess a Satvic type of mind, along with a healthy body. Size, or the lack of size, or great muscular strength is not necessary. On the other hand, qualities such as endurance, fortitude, temperament, memory, power of analysis, ability to concentrate and focus, capability to acknowledge, wisdom, intelligence, enthusiasm, discipline, attentiveness and carefulness, methodicalness, initiative, the ability to take on challenges, along with purity of body and heart, and good digestive powers are what it takes to cope with life. In Charaka's treatise, called "Rasayana Tantra", these qualities, and medication to enhance these, are dealt with in detail.

According to him, neglect of health owing to pre-occupation with one's occupation is also a contributor to the development of disease. This creates an imbalance in Doshas and the predominance of a particular Dosha, results in a chronic diseased condition. The treatment lies with restoring the predominant Dosha to a level of normality and providing a diet and mental stimulation that maintains equilibrium in the Doshas.

One particular medication for such conditions, especially in serious cases, is Abhaya (Embolic Myrobalans) with the pulp of Punarnava. One measure of Abhaya is mixed with four measures of the pulp of Punarnava and five measures of ghee and is boiled till the fluid content has completely evaporated. Then, an equal quantity of ghee is added along with an equal quantity of Vidari juice, with some pulp of Jeevanti, Bala and Atibala. To this is added, four times its volume of milk and its equal volume of Shatavari. This is then boiled till dry, and the procedure is repeated a hundred, or even a thousand times, depending upon the potency required, adding ghee every time. Finally, a measure of honey and sugar is added to this decoction, equal to a quarter of its weight. This, final medicine, is stored in a vessel made of material that will not react with it, usually of pure gold or silver. Earthen vessels may be used, but if so, the vessel should be first lined with ghee.

For the actual treatment, this must be administered to the patient in the manner of *Kutipraveshika*, which entails keeping the patient housebound in a room for days, even months, protected from the elements, wind and sunlight. The chamber in which the patient stays is an internal one, surrounded by other rooms whose doors and windows do not face each other. The patient first goes through a process of *Panchakarma*, which is a five-step body purifying process. The medicine is given twice daily with a diet of rice with milk or ghee and the dose is regulated to what the person can digest in ten hours. The administration continues until the person is sufficiently strong in physique and bulk, gaining as much weight as two and an eighth of his original and having imbibed as much as 512 tolas of the juice of Abhaya.

This ensures almost complete rejuvenation, slowing the aging process immensely, with substantial gain of memory, sexual prowess and immunity. These effects pass on to the patient's progeny as well, producing admirable, long-lived children, beautiful in appearance, strong and muscular, with bodies that function perfectly.

Charaka also dealt with the issue of those occupations that create the most risk to health of people pursuing them. These occupations have similar modern counterparts to which the analogy of Charaka can be extended. He found that the following type of people were always afflicted with disease:

Students of the Vedas: These people are prone to disease due to the intensity of effort and their neglect. They appear to have no time for their own physical welfare. There are many parallels in the modern world.

Servants of the King : Owing to regular and continuous performance to royal orders, such people have no time to attend to their own health, nor maintain healthy routines. They are dependant on the demands imposed on them by others higher up in the chain of command, and, surrounded by constant fear, which is not good for mental equilibrium as well. In the modern world, such demands on a worker are not limited to kings or royal personages, as employees in the consumer industries can testify.

Traders: People who are engaged in the work of continuously buying and selling, conducting transactions for money. Typically, such people are expected to stand or sit in one place for long periods of time.Neglect is the major factor for their developing disease.

Prostitutes : They are prone to all the infections that their customers carry, besides stress, neglect and not operating to healthy routines. Simply to appear attractive and to cater to their clients subjects them to stress and unhealthy applications.

Various forms of treatment exist for the above. The simplest may be the administration of an enema at night before going to bed and early in the morning, followed by a daily soak upto the neck for fifteen minutes, in a tub of water containing an emulsion of healing oils. Methods have been devised for such treatment in standing and prone positions. A healthy diet is a treatment in itself – a diet rich in milk, ghee, butter-milk, variety of fruits, vegetables and spotted grains.

People are advised to consider their choice of livelihood. Is it compatible with their health? Is it possible to bring beneficial change to their method of livelihood? People are also advised to ponder over the mental aspects of health, on aspects of their occupation that impinge on mental balance. After all, good health is essential to happiness and for the pursuit of one's very livelihood.

# 20

# PUBLIC HEALTH

The community as a whole, without regard to class, caste, creed or colour, constitutes the public. The one thing all members of any community have in common is that they have come together for the purpose of living, and are inter-dependant on each other. If the survival of the community is threatened, so is the personal survival of individual members. Yet, it is impossible for any community of any significant size to consist entirely of healthy members. Some, who are healthy at one point of time, may be unhealthy at others. Some may be chronically unhealthy; while the sheer numbers that constitute a community can itself create unhygienic conditions that threaten health within. Public Health is the generic term that applies to addressing the health needs of a community and the intention of Public Swasthavritta is to attain and maintain its healthy condition. Thus, it embraces the issues of supplying pure water, material for good food, such as milk and victuals, ventilation in the construction of dwelling places and a system for the disposal of the waste that is a consequent of large clusters of population. It must also embrace issues of other essential supplies, attention to the matter of protection for its members from acts of aggression, and, the generation of employment for its members.

It is, therefore, the duty of every individual member to contribute, to the extent possible, to the welfare of one's community. One should help the poor, diseased, disabled and the miserable. Drawing upon the Swasthavritta of yore, it was said that it is the duty of an individual to treat even an ant as one would treat another. One must respect God, the king (read administration), elders, the cow, brahmins and physicians. One should give alms to beggars and do good to one's opposers, avoiding grudges and acts which can create enmity, such as designating someone as an enemy or betraying confidentiality. One must follow public convention. One must develop the capacity for compassion, even for animals and the poor. One must control one's own deeds and thoughts and assist others in the discharge of their duties and obligations.

Further, Manusmriti, Chanakya's Arthashastra – which has dealt extensively on matters of public health, and the Bhagavad Geeta, have this to add – One must help another in procuring food, develop the spirit of cooperation, distribution of assets and for securing health and happiness. The king (the government) must protect his subject (the people) in all respects, arranging for the supply of their needs. Good people rejoice in the happiness of their friends and fellowmen and the king should be satisfied only when all his subjects are happy. Orphans, underprivileged children, the insane, the ill and the old were all identified as sections of the community which deserved special help. Thoughtless acts of waste disposal, such as throwing rubbish on the roads, were punished, as were acts of ablution in zones prohibited for such acts, designated holy places, reservoirs, waterways, lakes, public places and offices. Care was to be exercised for disposal of the dead, whether human or animal, whether pet or beast of burden. They could not be disposed off just anywhere. Punishment for violation usually consisted of a series of progressively heavier fines.

Inspectors were instituted by the government for regularly inspecting the state of water-bodies, including rivers and lakes, and every river was supposed to be provided with a bridge over it for the convenience of the public. Every village was provided with at least a temple and a garden for public use. Calamities such as famine, drought, flood, fires that led to epidemics occurred during Chanakya's time, and he studied all of them in order to find measures for remedy and containment. Accordingly, measures against fires breaking out became mandatory. A house was required to keep in readiness, five vessels of water, a ladder, a pair of tongs and a leather bag for carrying water. Thatched roofs came to be prohibited and a larger quantity of water stored at planned places for use by the community in case of a fire of severe proportions. Plans were drawn up for coping with floods. People in low lying places were given directions to earmarked, safer locations on higher ground. Appeals were sent out to the public for assistance to the worst hit.

Meanwhile, a system for controlling disease was also instituted. While a cadre of physicians were trained to fight disease, a cadre of spirituals, in the form of *Siddhas* and *Tapasvis*, were set up to offer propiation to the Gods. Reserves of grain and a public distribution system was created for use in emergency. The better off were taxed so that the funds thus collected would constitute a pool to be used for purchase of grain and essentials from other communities and governments, when required after natural calamity and during epidemics. Plantation was often used as a form of protection in places situated near threatening tracts of water.

Animals were often a source of epidemic level infection, sometimes after infected flesh was consumed and it was realised that rotting carcasses in the forests were a potential source. Various methods were employed to contain this, including poisoning. The juice of the Snuhi tree was coated on corn as bait for culling rodents, while extracts of Mandana was used to poison predators like the tiger.

Steps to protect people from crime were instituted by the government of the time and the king, as a leader, was constituted mainly to provide a uniform chain of command for fighting off invasion. War, it was realised, is a grave threat to the health of a community and ethical principles, which composed *Dharmayuddha*, were structured for fighting war. Those who did not follow these principles were termed barbarians.

# 21

# HEALTH FOR THE MILITARY

The military guards a nation's people, property and territory, and was constituted as larger communities bonded together under a common leader, the king. The primary reason for constituting the military was to protect against aggression and to defend. Military Swasthavritta was given attention as an important part of public Swasthavritta, since soldiers are drawn from the public and return to it when their soldiering is over. The nature of their duties demands that military personnel be extremely healthy and that this state be preserved properly and efficiently, and so was the subject of much study and analysis. By employing youth, in the prime of health, full of energy, with powers of sustenance and resistance, the health of the military was easily maintained. It was not the practise of those times to employ permanent armies, though a minimal permanent force was kept for the personal protection of the king. Youth from agricultural occupations were drafted after a national call was issued when war threatened.

The health of the king was of prime importance, with lesser importance given to the health of the lower ranks. Again, Chanakya is a major source of insights into the practices of those times. These employed methods of warfare such as setting fires to crops, attacks on food and supply chains, transporting water and methods of poisoning. Whole studies were devoted to the subject of poison warfare, from poisoning food for entire armies and populaces, to poisoned jewels to kill select leaders and the employment of poisoned arrows and weapons. Even black art was employed to sap the vitality of opposing armies.

The king employed his dedicated physician(s) for protecting him from threats whose source could be food, drink or jewels or simply disease. The physician was chosen for his proficiency in medicine and knowledge of disease, both practical and theoretical, coupled with whether he was trustworthy and of good character. Further, he had to possess a good temperament and capabilities of being a source of inspiration. Obviously, someone with a formidable reputation, capable of clever handling of issues of statecraft. Such a physician was also expected to provide medical solutions for the problems of the realm, to cope with epidemics, the aftermath of storms, floods, drought, natural and man-made calamities. Not the least of these would present as seasonal disturbances and pollution of the air and water, times of poor harvests and famine, infestation and contagion. He was also expected to cope with the other world, with the evil spirits who were believed to behind natural calamity.

A method of treatment that evolved during those times involved treating the king with *Sneha*, both externally and internally, along with *Swedana*, a process of inducing perspiration. This was followed with *Basthividhi*, the administration of a medicated enema, which provides nutrition while cleansing. This legacy forms a part of Panchakarma therapy, detailed by the author in his book "*Panchakarma Treatment of Ayurveda*". Other methods have been *Vamana* (induced vomiting), *Virechana* (induced purgation) and *Nasya*.

This line of treatment not only cures, but is also both prophylactic and rejuvenating for those who do not suffer from disease. Another therapy developed by the physicians of those days is *Rasayana* therapy, based on nutrient intake. For Royalty, physicians resorted to *Acharya Rasayana,* for which, according to Charaka, the person must first be truthful, compassionate, in control of his mind, detached from passions, helpful to others, dutiful, celibate, studious about the scriptures and teachings of the great, and should have performed for the benefit of country and community. Reading from the *Dharmashastra* and the works of the *Maharishis* are specified by Charaka, and examples of people worthy of Acharya Rasayana in more recent times can be Jawaharlal Nehru and Mahatma Gandhi. The responsibility of protecting people of stature lay with the king, who had the charge of testing food served from the royal kitchen.

Military staff were at risk from poisoning by seductresses and the physician was responsible for providing them adequate protection, and conducting tests on food, drink, victuals, applications like oils and cleaners, ornaments, clothes and covering, apparatus and medication, all of which were potential carriers of poisons. Animals were employed to signal the presence of poison. The effect of edibles on crows and flies were observed, their death signaling the obvious. The *Chakora* bird, it was believed, would change the colour of its eyes when sensing poison. Likewise, it was believed that the *Kokila* would change its tone of voice, the *Krauncha* bird would faint, the Peacock would dance, while apes would pass motion and *Hamsas* start screeching, in the presence of poison. A modern parallel is the use of canaries in coal mines; canaries being able to smell methane at levels far below human sensory thresholds. Notwithstanding the above, Chanakya had researched the issue of poisoning thoroughly and had prepared exhaustive lists on their types, effects, symptoms, detection and antidotes. Charaka and Sushrutha contributed further.

# 22

# PREVENTION OF DISEASE

Roganuthpadaniyam has been a major source in Ayurveda for the prevention of disease. By stopping a disease from occurring in the first place, one prevents it. Simple measures that make up Sadvritta, like brushing teeth, bathing and cleaning are effective, as dealt with earlier in this book. Then, there are the 'regimen' measures, daily as well as seasonal, which have also been detailed earlier.

Next comes the issue of suppression of natural urges, passing urine or faeces, flatus, hunger, thirst, sneezing, yawning, shedding tears, vomiting, ejaculation, respiration, rest and the like. Suppression of these makes the individual liable to disease whether by the person's own control or by obstruction or medicine. The control of urges, thus, can be either natural or unnatural.

Unnatural control or delay of urges may occur because of constraints of time and place and because of work. Obstructions, when they occur in the passages within the body, are instances of natural suppression.

There are thirteen natural urges in the body consisting of passing *Adhovata* (flatus), passing Mala (faeces), passing Mutra (urine), *Kshawathu* (sneeze), *Trishna* (thirst), *Kshudha* (hunger), *Nidra* (sleep), *Kasa* (cough), *Swasa* (shortness of breath), *Jrumbha* (yawn), *Asru* (tears), *Chardhi* (vomit) and Shukra (semen).

The *Apanavayu* (flatus) controls the ejection of Shukra (semen), *Arthava* (ovum), Shakruth (bowels) and Mutra (urine), and so, it needs to be in a healthy state. Vata works in a way to encourage excretion from the body, and if natural urges are suppressed, Vata will become aggravated and work in any manner it deems fit to force expulsion. Aggravated Vata will produce disease.

Symptoms of obstruction of Apnavayu are Gulma (fantom tumour), Udvarta (belching, accompanied with constipation or diarrhoea and pain in the abdomen), retention of excreta, loss of vision or weakness in the sensory organs, digestive disorders and heart disease. Treatment for the above consists of taking an ounce of castor-oil with a tablespoonful of milk, at bedtime, for a week.

When the natural urge for evacuating the bowels is suppressed, the symptoms that result, usually are, pain in the calf muscles, cold, headache, belching, piercing pains in the stomach, feeling of obstruction and pain in the chest, vomiting, Gulma, Udvarta. Treatment for the above consists of taking five grams of *Triphala* at bedtime or the administration of oily enemas for a few days, and a diet that facilitates the normal movement of Vata.

Suppression of passage of urine leads to pain, urinary calculi, pain in the bladder or in the vagina or penis, or in the region of the groin, and eventually, Gulma and Udvarta.

Suppositories in the anus help the expulsion of flatus and faecal matter. Soaking in a tub, sudation and medication to clear the bowels also help. Typically, such medication consists of a dose of one ounce of *Abhayarista* with a gram of Triphala powder after food, along with, between 20 and 30 ml. of pure ghee from a cow, before and after a meal.

Suppression of belching will lead to feelings of tastelessness, gripping pains in the trunk and stomach region.

Suppression of sneezing will lead to ringing in the head, loss of function in the eyes and ears, and loss of smell. This can be treated with medicated smoking, collyrium and errhine. Suppression of thirst will lead to consumption, wasting of the body, indigestion, deafness, giddiness and pain in the heart.

While the natural physical urges are not to be suppressed, humans are subject to a variety of mental urges as well. To name a few – *Irshya* (hatred), *Dwesha* (prejudice), *Matsarya* (vengeance). These mental feelings and urges require to be controlled as they vitiate the Vata, leading to disease. These are controlled through developing positive aspects of the mind such as *Dheer* (calm), *Dhairya* (patience) and *Atmadi Vijnana* (knowledge of the soul). This is easier said than done though, as the conditions are produced due to the vitiation of Vata. The subject is dealt with in detail in Chapter 4 of the *Astanga Hridaya Sutrasthana of Vagbhata.*

People who control their natural urges, usually have a lean and emaciated appearance and are prone to feeling thirsty, vomiting and pain. Lines of treatment for them can be Snehana (oleation), Swedana and Basthividhi, the administration of a medicated enema. Prayer, meditation and Pranayana are all helpful in maintaining a balanced state of mind and in keeping the brain in equilibrium.

# 23

# MAINTAINING HEALTH STATISTICS

The National Health Services have been created for the purpose of dealing with health related matters and subjects. Information needs to be collected and collated.in order to examine for analysis, for research and training, for planning and implementation. Organisations within the umbrella provided by the National Health Services have the responsibility for such collection.

Data is collected –
1. On a demographic basis i.e. based on the population
2. Based on the problems of an area or populace
3. Based on particular diseases, their investigation and treatment

This data is then collated in the form of charts, tables and percentages.

Data comprises of –
1. Demographic details, such as locations and characteristics
2. Health statistics involving state of health, mortality, age medians and such
3. Resources, such as beds, workers, doctors, surgeons etc.
4. Utility of health services – attendance of patients, patients awaiting admission
5. Quality of health services
6. Economic details – funds allocation, collections and expenditure

## Utility of Health Information

1. What is available by way of health services, how much availed
2. Benchmarking – comparison of standards at the local, national and international levels
3. Planning, administration and proper maintenance of services
4. Propriety of service – who does it reach, is it fit for its target
5. Identifying areas for research
6. Identifying its beneficiaries

## Basic Health Information

1. Census: conducted once in ten years in India
2. Registration: birth, death, marriage of every individual; adoption, divorce. In India, this is per the Central Birth & Death Registration Act of 1969.
3. Notifications: such as those on disease
4. Hospital records
5. Hospital registers of disease
6. Linking records
7. Epidemilogical surveillance
8. Records of different agencies in Health
9. Environmental data
10. Manpower statistics
11. Population surveys

## Methods of keeping statistics

| | |
|---|---|
| Tabulation | - tables |
| Charts | - pie charts, bar charts |
| Diagrams | - line diagrams, graphs |
| Maps | - static, GIS |

Statistics can be kept by age, frequency, as averages, mean and medians, by distribution (normal and standard deviation).

# 24

# MODERN NUTRITION

Nutrition is intrinsic to life, for its growth and maintenance, and the foods that supply the body can be classified as:
1. Energy yielding foods
2. Body building foods
3. Protective foods
All three classes are required by the body in a balanced way.

The make-up of the human body is approximately 17% protein, 12% fats, 7% minerals, 1% carbohydrate and a large amount of water. Foods must replenish all of these. Ghee, for example, is the Ayurvedic equivalent for fat. Dal is the equivalent for protein, while rice, milk and egg supply combinations of carbohydrates, protein and fat.

**Proteins** are the basic building blocks of the human body and consist of carbon, hydrogen, oxygen, nitrogen, sulphur, phosphorous and iron. Proteins are vital for the growth of the body and to replenish wear and tear. Protein is the basic matter that makes up all tissue such as muscle, as well as blood, antibodies, plasma, haemoglobin, enzymes and hormones.

Proteins also have a protective role; manufacture of phagocytes, for example, requires protein. Amino acids, in turn, are the basic building blocks for proteins, and some examples are leucin, isoleucine, methionine, phenylaravine, tryptophane, valine and histidine. Milk, egg, fish and meat are all rich sources of protein for the non-vegetarian, while gram, seeds, beans and dal are sources for protein for vegetarians.

As a thumb rule, the daily intake of protein should be one gram of protein per kilogram of body weight plus 10grams. Thus, a man weighing 45 kilos for example, requires to ingest in the region of 55 grams of protein a day to maintain health, while a woman weighing 35 kilos requires to ingest 45 grams a day. Lower intake will lead to wasting diseases such as Marasmus and Kwashiorkar. Pregnant women require between 14 to 25 grams more.

However, different sources of protein differ in both the quantity and the quality of protein they supply to the body when eaten. Foods that supply protein are evaluated by way of their –

1. Digestible coefficient (D.C.)

2. Biological value (B.V.)

3. Protein efficiency ratio

4. Use of net protein (N.P.U.)

A comparative table of different sources of protein is produced at the end of this chapter.

| Infants and Children | | Quantity required |
|---|---|---|
| 1. 1 to 3 months | Milk | 2.3 gms |
| 2. 3 to 6 months | Milk | 1.8 gms |
| 3. 6 to 9 months | Milk + Vegetables | 1.8 gms |
| 4. 9 to 12 months | Milk + Vegetables | 1.5 gms |
| 5. 1 to 3 years | 1.83 gm/kg bodyweight | 22 gms |
| 6. 4 to 6 years | 1.56 gm/kg bodyweight | 20 gms |
| 7. 7 to 9 years | 1.35 gm/kg bodyweight | 36 gms |

| Male Adolescents | | |
|---|---|---|
| 1. 10 to 12 years | 1.24 gm/kg bodyweight | 43 gms |
| 2. 13 to 15 years | 1.10 gm/kg bodyweight | 52 gms |
| 3. 16 to 18 years | 0.94 gm/kg bodyweight | 53 gms |

| Female Adolescents | | |
|---|---|---|
| 1. 10 to 12 years | 1.17 gm/kg bodyweight | 43 gms |
| 2. 13 to 15 years | 0.95 gm/kg bodyweight | 43 gms |
| 3. 16 to 18 years | 0.88 gm/kg bodyweight | 44 gms |

Lack of protein leads to conditions such as anaemia, ansarca (general swelling of the body), being underweight, wasting, diarrhoea, lethargy and lassitude, fatigue and to wounds not healing.

**Fats** are also essential for the body. Besides providing cushioning for the organs, fats are a source of energy, one gram of fat containing nine kilocalories. They also assist in absorbing vitamins A, D and E and in the functions of the heart, intestines and kidneys. Meat and oils, both animal and vegetable oils, are rich sources of fat. Examples of sources of fat from animals are ghee, butter, fish liver oils, cod liver oil and fish oils, while examples of sources of fat from vegetables are groundnut oil, til oil, cottonseed oil and sunflower oil. Major deficiency in fat can also lead to skin conditions like pronoderma (thikening of skin).

**Carbohydrates** are the immediate supplier of energy to the cells of the body. Sugars such as glucose, galactose and fructose, starches such as cereals, millets, roots, and vegetables like potatoes are sources of carbohydrate. Starchy foods such as cereals and millets and fibrous fruits are a source of cellulose and roughage, which is essential for the bowel movement. Lack of roughage produces constipation and can lead to conditions such as cancer of the colon, arteriosclerosis, heart disease, appendicitis and gallstones.

**Vitamins** are another essential nutrient required by the body for the growth of bones and the skin, functioning of the mucus membrane and to prevent diseases. Vitamin A is essential for the skin, Vitamin D is essential for healthy bone formation, Vitamin E for the heart and blood, and lack of it during pregnancy can lead to abortion. Lack of Vitamin K leads to loss of the clotting function in blood. Rich sources of vitamins include liver, butter, eggs, milk, carrots, pumpkins and fruits. Mangoes and papayas are fruits which are abundant in all the main vitamins.

The daily requirement of vitamin is – about 750 micrograms of Vitamin A for adolescents and adults, though women after delivery need an additional 400 micrograms. Infants require even less, about 400 micrograms daily. 15 milligrams of Vitamin E, and between 1 and 2 milligrams of Vitamin K are required daily. 0.5 milligrams of Thiomine and 0.6 milligrams of Riboflavin are required per 1000 KCal. of energy expended. Thiomine is available in fish oils, oilseeds, meat, eggs and vegetables. Rice, before milling, is a great source of Riboflavin, but because most of the rice that we consume is of the milled kind, supplements by way of tablets or injections are often needed. Liver, milk, eggs, meat and dals are all good sources of Riboflavin.

|  | Protein | D.C. | B.V. | NPU |
|---|---|---|---|---|
|  | % | % | % | % |
| **Animal Foods** |  |  |  |  |
| 1. Eggs | 13.3 | 98 | 98 | 96 |
| 2. Cow's milk | 3.5 | 95 | 85 | 81 |
| 3. Meat | 19.8 | 96 | 82 | 79 |
| 4. Fish | 21.5 | 96 | 80 | 77 |
|  |  |  |  |  |
| **Cereal** |  |  |  |  |
| 1. Wheat | 11.8 | 85 | 60 | 51 |
| 2. Milled Rice | 7 | 93 | 70 | 65 |
| 3. Maize | 11.1 | 85 | 50 | 43 |
|  |  |  |  |  |
| **Gram** |  |  |  |  |
| 1. Bengal gram(Chana) | 22.5 | 84 | 62 | 52 |
| 2. Black gram (Urad) | 24 | 82 | 54 | 45 |
| 3. Green gram(Moong) | 24 | 85 | 58 | 49 |
| 4. Red gram (TuvarDal) | 22.3 | 83 | 56 | 46 |
|  |  |  |  |  |
| **Seeds and Oilseeds** |  |  |  |  |
| 1. Chana | 26.7 | 92 | 54 | 50 |
| 2. Coconut | 4.5 | 82 | 67 | 56 |
| 3. Soyabean | 40 | 86 | 64 | 55 |
| 4. Til | 18.3 | 80 | 60 | 48 |

# 25

# SAMSHODHANA AND SAMSHAMANA

Oleation, Sweating and blood-letting are some of the techniques employed in Panchakarma therapy and briefly detailed below.

*Snehana Karma* or oleation is a part of *Poorva Karma* which is to be conducted before initiating Panchakarma therapy. This dissolves and rids the body of the toxins present in it (a process known as *Vishyandana*) and it also produces softness or sleekness in the body versus hardness or boniness (known as *Mridutva* and *Kledana Karma*). While small modifications in diet – simply a larger intake of fats during the Sharad Ritu or season, a larger intake of Vasa and Majja during Vasanta, and Taila during Pravrita are sufficient, Sneha Pana (the actual act of drinking oils or fats) may become necessary during summer and in cases when the Vata and Pitta doshas are aggravated during the night-time. For cases of excessive Kapha Doshas during the cold season, Sneha Pana during the day is also beneficial. In such cases, the patient should drink only hot water whilst on treatment. Sneha Pana is administrated in doses which vary from the maximum, that which takes twenty-four hours to digest; to the medium, which takes twelve hours to digest; to the minimum, that takes six hours to digest.

Sneha Pana is good for sweda-indicated patients, those with a rough body, alcoholics and the sexually hyperactive. It improves the flatus, *Vatanulomana*, and produces oily stools, increases digestive fire and makes for a soft body. It should not be administered to those who require dry treatment, those with Kapha and obesity, those who salivate excessively, or suffer from diarrhoea, dryness of throat, thirst, anorexia, distaste for food, abdominal disorders and vomiting. It should not be administered to those in a coma or those on vasti and Nasya treatment, nor in cases of poisoning and the weak.

*Swedana Karma* or Sudation Therapy is a treatment that makes the body perspire and thus removes morbid material from it. This form of treatment is generally employed after the patient has undergone oleation, and there are two broad classes of Swedana Karma. *Agni Sweda* uses fire as a medium for inducing sweat, while *Niragni Sweda* uses means other than fire. The purpose of both forms is to remove morbid material from the body, from the *shaakha* or the bloodstream (the *raktadhaya dhatava twak cha*) to the koshta or the alimentary tract. Further sub-classification of Sweda includes:

1. S*aagni Sweda / Anagni Sweda*

2. *Ekaanga* or localised *Sweda / Sarvanga* or whole body *Sweda*

3. S*nigdha* (oil-based) *Sweda / Rooksha* (dry) *Sweda*

4. Sweda customised for the seasons (*Ritu*) and with varying potency (*Bal*) such as *Mahan, Madhyama* and *Hraswa*

5. Sweda with varying methods of application, namely *Taapa, Ushna, Upanaha* and *Pravara*

6. *Shamshaneeya Sweda* and *Samsodhananga Sweda*

These classes of treatment are based upon different principles and usage. Sweda is generally useful in disorders of the Kapha and Vata, and because of employment of heat (*Ushna*) and pungency (*Teekshana*), it vitiates Pitta. There are thirteen types of Sweda which may be administered in any of the classes given above and these are listed as under:

1. *Sankara*
2. *Prasthara*
3. *Nadi*
4. *Parisheka*
5. *Avgaha*
6. *Jentaka*
7. *Ashmaghana*
8. *Karshu*
9. *Kuti*
10. *Kupa*
11. *Kumbhi*
12. *Bhu*
13. *Holaka*

Sudation therapy benefits the following types of people:

1. Those with Vata Pradhana diseases – the nervous
2. Those with Kapha Pradhana diseases – the withdrawn
3. Those who are being prepared for Samsodhana or purification therapy
4. Those who are being prepared for surgery

The benefits of Sudation therapy are:

1. Control of obesity
2. Regulation of the body weight and size
3. Produces a sleekness in the body and tones it up
4. Rids the body of stiffness
5. Improves skin tone

6. Produces suppleness in the joints
7. Improves resistance to cold
8. Liquifies the Doshas
9. Regulates the Vatas
10. Improves digestion
11. Purifies the Srotas
12. Removes lassitude
13. Promotes perspiration, thereby ridding the body of toxins

*Vamana Karma* or Emesis Therapy is the first step of Panchakarma and the best treatment for disorders of the Kapha. It is also known as Chardana, Nissharana and Abhisyandana, and regulates the Doshas of the upper body by removing the vitiated one from the bloodstream to the shukra and to the the gastro-intestinal tract. Quoting from Charaka (1-4) *"Tatra Dosha Haranam Urdhwa Bhaga Vamana Sanjna Kam,"* meaning that there are six kinds of emetics – the hot, the acute, the subtle, the spreading (*Vikasi*), the *Vyavayi* and the *Urdhwa Bhaga Prabhava.*

Vamana is unsuitable for the very obese, the highly emaciated, the very young and the very old, and those who are in advanced stages of weakness, exhaustion, illness, such as tuberculosis or starvation. It is unsuitable during fasting and after exercise, such as after lifting heavy weights, after coitus and during periods of focused study.

*Virechana Karma* or Purgation Therapy is the second step of Panchakarma and the best treatment for disorders of the Pitta. Oleation and sudation treatment, in conjunction with purgation, is employed here. This rids the body of the Doshas through the bowels or *Gudamarga*. Some of the relevant quotes regarding the procedure have been *"Tatra Dosha Haranam Adhobhagam Virechana Sanjna Kam"*(Charaka K, 1-4), **"Virechanam Sanjnakam"** (Charaka Sutra 25/40), and from the Astaanga Sangraha Sutra 27, opining that it should be the treatment of choice for disorders of the Pitta and Kapha.

Therapies may be based upon the use of mild purgatives or laxatives called *Mriduvirechakas,* such as Aragwadha, or upon the use of medium-level purgatives or laxatives called *Madhyamavirechakas* such as Trivrit, or upon the use of drastic purgatives or laxatives called *Teekshana-virechakas* such as Snuhi. Treatment can be of the *Anulomana* kind employing Haritaki or of the *Samsrana* kind employing Aragwadha. It may be of either the Snigdha or oil-based kind or the Rooksha or dry kind.

Virechana Karma benefits the following types of people:

1. Those with Pitta Pradhana diseases – anaemia (*Paandu*), jaundice (*Kaamala*)

2. Those with blood diseases – leprosy, many skin diseases, haemorrhagic diathesis (*Rakta Pitta*), abscesses, cancers and *Arbuda*

3. Those with *Shodhana Pradhana Vyaadhis* – Udvarta, intestinal worms (*Krimikoshta*) and constipation

4. Those with Pitta Adhistana diseases – fever, heart disease (*Hridroga*) and jaundice (*Kaamala*)

A detailed treatise by the author, titled *Panchakarma Treatment of Ayurveda* is available in English, Hindi and Kannada for those who want to study this form of treatment in greater depth.

Proper Virechana will lead to feelings of relief, "Indriyas will be delighted", lightness in the body, increased digestive fire, improvement in first stools followed by Pitta and bile. Only the vitiated kapha and vata are removed and signs of flatus and Ayoga are absent.

**Symptoms of Virechana Shuddhi**

| | Symptoms of | Pravara Shodhana | Madhyama Shodhana | Heena Shodhana |
|---|---|---|---|---|
| A. | Vaigiki Shuddhi | 30 ovegas | 20 ovegas | 10 ovegas |
| B. | Maanaki Shuddhi | 4 prasthas | 3 prasthas | 2 prasthas |
| C. | Antaki Shuddhi Virechana | Kaphanta Virechana | Kaphanta Virechana | Kaphanta |

*Vasti Karma* or Enema Therapy is the third step of Panchakarma and the best treatment for disorders of the Vata, striking at its root, the large intestine or *Pakwashya*. Enema is administered using the bladder of animals and consists of four classes, depending on the organ being treated, namely:

1. **Pakwashyagata** (for the large intestine)
2. **Garbhashyagata** (for the uterus)
3. **Mutrashyagata** (for the bladder)
4. **Vranagata** (for wounds and ulcers)

Vasti Karma will provide the following benefits:

1. It alleviates the Doshas.
2. It helps with the formation of proper stools (Malas).
3. It balances the structure of the body towards proper proportions – the skinny will put on flesh while the obese will shed some.

4. It will improve vision and brighten the eyes.

5. It will enhance longevity.

6. It acts as a health protector.

7. It stops hair loss and alopecia.

8. It balances the Tridoshas

9. It wards off diseases of the body and mind.

Depending upon the drugs employed, it may be:
1. Niruha or Asthaapana Vasti
2. Anuvasana Vasti of either the Sneha or Maatra kinds

It may be further be classified depending upon the number of repetitions, which are typically as under:

1. Karmavasti – 12 Niruha + 18 Anuvasana, totalling 30 doses.

2. Kalavasti – 6 Niruha + 10 Anuvasana, totalling 16 doses.

3. Yogavasti – 3 Niruha + 5 Anuvasana, totalling 8 doses.

Asthaapana Vasti is helpful for conditions involving Vata, Mutra or urine, semen, diarrhoea, belching. Fantom tumours, abdominal pains, timira, (eyedisease) obstruction of faeces, headaches and migraine, paralysis including facial ones, strokes, convulsions, shoulder pain, stiffness of the neck and jaw, diseases of the nervous system, and for those who will undergo Shodhana. Anuvasana Vasti is helpful for Vata conditions and controlling excessive appetites. As above, the two are used in conjunction.

Vasti treatment is contraindicated for the pregnant, the comatose, the dyspnoeic and the anaemic. It is also not for those who are suffering from enlargement of the spleen, gastroenteritis, diarrhoea, Amadoshas, Prameha, skin disease and haemorrhoids.

*Nasya Karma* or Errhine Therapy, also known as Nasal insufflation, is a treatment which employs the nasal passage for administering medicines, usually oil-based, called Snehas. Also known as Sirovirechana and Murdhavirechana, it has been mentioned in the scriptures – "*Nasyam Bhavan Nasyam*" and "*Nasahi Sirasodwaram*" (Astanga Hridaya Sutra 20/1).

There are five different methods of Nasya, namely:

1. Navana – either Snehana or Samsodhana
2. Avapeedana – either Samsodhana or Sthambana
3. Dhumrapana
4. Dhooma – either Prayogika Vairchanika or Snehika
5. Pratimansa – either Snehana or Virechana

Nasya may be classified by its three functions, and may be either **Rechana** or **Tarpana** or **Shamana**. An alternate system of classification is according to drugs used for treatment, and under this system, it can employ either *Phal* (fruit), *Mula* (root), *Patra* (leaf), *Kanda* (bark), *Twak* (skin), *Niryaasa* (extract) or *Paya* (milk).

Samyak Shuddhi of Nasya is invariably to be followed by consumption of taila for Vata and ghee for Pitta.

The benefits of Nasya include – lightness of the body, improved sleep, alleviation of disease specially those of the sensory organs, clearing the head and purification of the Srota.

A technique widely employed during the times of Sushrutha for Sodhana therapy was *Raktamokshana* or blood-letting. This was classified by method and function. Methods employed were by *Shastra* (using an instrument to draw blood), with *Prachaana* (induced bleeding) and *Siryavyadha* (by cutting a vein). The purposes would be *Sringavacharana* for controlling Vatadushti, *Jalaukavacharana* or leeching for controlling Pitttadushti, *Alaabuvavacharana* for controlling Kaphadushti, *Ghatiyantra* for controlling combinations of Kaphadushti and Vatadushti. Raktamokshana was supposed to improve the clarity of body and mind, digestive fires, strength and as a treatment for blood disorders.

# 26

# RASAYANA AND VAJEEKARANA

Among the eight forms of *Chikitsa* or modes of treatment recognised in Ayurveda as alleviators of disease, and health, two promoters happen to be Rasayana and Vajeekarana. Rasayana happens to be the term for tonic and is derived from Rasa, which means nutrient. The scriptures say "*Labhopayehi Shasthanam Rasadinam Rasayanam*" – that in order to be healthy, it is imperative for man to have proper nutrition for his tissues and Dhatus. Special nutrition, by way of tonics, produce vigour in life and a long life, besides *Vyaadhi Kshmata* (resistance to disease).

Rasayana can be of two types – tonics for the tissues and tonics for the brain and mental equilibrium or stimulation. The latter are called *Medhya rasayana* or tranquilisers and together with Vajeekarana drugs work as antidepressants by stimulating brain cells.

Rasayanas meant for the nutrition of the body, the first type, is further classified as either:

1. *Rasavardhaka Rasayana*, which provides nutrition for tissue matter, substances such as Shatavari, Kharjoora, milk and ghee.

2. *Agnivardhaka Rasayana*, which also provides tissue nutrition, but with the additional benefit of being promoters of digestion, such as Pippali or piper longum.

3. *Sroto Shodhakara Rasayana* such as Guggulu, which produce *Sroto Shodhaka* or improvements in the circulatory system.

4. *Naimithika Rasayana,* which deals with cures for a diseased condition and with substances that have a prophylactic action. Examples include Triphala for eye disease, Tuwaraka for skin disease, Shatavari, Jyotishmathi and Yastimadhu for heart disease.

In Ayurveda, regimes of treatment have evolved over the years based on the administration of tonics and how to get the most benefit from them. These regimes can be either *Vaatapika*, meaning treatment outdoors, or *Kutipraveshika*, meaning treatment indoors. There are five specialised branches of Rasayana, namely –

1. *Poshakarasa* – dealing with the subject of nutrition in general.

2. *Agni* – dealing with the subject of 'digestive fire' through its two respective sub-branches, *Deepana* which focuses on issues relating to digestion and *Pachana*, which focuses on issues relating to assimilation.

3. *Srotas* – dealing with the circulatory system.

4. *Dheerghaayu Vyadeshmatava* – dealing with issues of soothing, calming and recovery from illness.

5. *Medha* – as referred to earlier in the text, this deals with tonics for the intellect and the brain.

*Achara Rasayana,* is the term for the special regime of Rasayana reserved for, and known to be beneficial to only those who have achieved a Satvic state.

## A List of Some Tonics Commonly Employed in Ayurvedic treatments

As Brain Tonics (*Medha Rasayana*): Shankhapushpi, Brahmi

For Eye Diseases (*Naimithika Rasayana*): Triphala, Shatavari, Jyotishmati, Yastimadhu

For Heart Disease (*Hridroga*): Shaliparni, Arjun, Tuwaraka (for *Twak*)

For Tuberculosis (*Amavata*): Arjun, Garlic

For Rheumatoid Arthritis (also a form of *Amavata*): Amritavalli (Tinospora Cordifolia), Bhallataka (Semicarpusanacardium)

For Nervous Disorders (*Vatavyadhi*): Guggulu (Comminphora Mukul), Bala (Sida Cordifolia)

For Infections of the Urinary Tract (*Prameha*): Shilajit, Amalaki

For Obesity (*Medoroga*): Guggulu, Haritaki

For Blood Purification (*Rakta Vata*): Garlic, Bala, Rasna

For High Blood Pressure (*Rakta Chapa*): Kasturi, Kupeelu

For Urticaria (*Shita Pitta*): Haridra (Curcuma Longo)

For Skin Disease (*Kusta*): Khadira (Acacia Catechu)

To improve Circulation (*Srota Rasayana*): Pippali, Bhallataka, Garlic

To improve Digestion (*Agni Rasayana*): Vidanga (Embelia ribes), Haritaki, Pippali, Gold Bhasma, Makaradwaja, Abhraka Bhasma

For *Dhaatwaagni Rasayana:* Amalaki, Guduchi, Kumari (Aloes)

Whole regimes have developed around some of these herbs and natural extracts and some of the prominent ones are – Amalaki Rasayana, Triphala Rasayana, Aswagandha Rasayana, Bhallataka Rasayana, Shilajit Rasayana and Brahma Rasayana. These are known as the *Yogas of Rasayana*.

**Vajeekarana (Therapy to improve virility)** – Great importance was given in early times to therapies that involved virility as the propagation of the race depended on it. Thus it was postulated that the four essential needs of mankind, namely, Dharma or spirituality, Artha or wealth, Kama or the sexual pleasures, and Moksha or salvation could only be attained by a person healthy in every way, physically, mentally, socially and economically. Because nutrition and nutritional supplements play an important part in achieving such a state of health, the study of Vajeekara foods was an important subject in Ayurveda. Studies involved every aspect such as virility or *Vaj*, potency or *Veerya*, stamina, stimulants and aphrodisiacs, and cures for sexually transmitted disease. Such foods are recommended for all normal, healthy people, the young as well as the middle-aged.

*Vajeekara Yoga* is the term for the regimes that benefit sexual performance or are used for the treatment of sexual dysfunction and disease. These are –

1. Apathykara swarasa
2. Kamalalakshadichoorna
3. Vanarigutika
4. Mahachandanadi tablets and Taila
5. Dashamularistam
6. Kaminividrvana Rasa
7. Puspadhanvarasa
8. Chandrodaya Rasa
9. Vasanta Kusumakara Rasa

10. Makaradwaja
11. Kamadeva Ghrita
12. Jayamangala Rasa
13. Narasimha Choorna
14. Amrita Choorna

However before resorting to any of these therapies, it is required to first carry out a Panchakarma purification.

Foods that are either astringent, bitter, pungent, very hot, or too salty, sour and alkaline – are not compatible with Vajeekarana therapy.

Vajeekara drugs act upon the production of Catecholamines and thus act as antidepressants and mood elevators. They are, thus, quite useful in treating mental disorders and promoting tranquility of mind.

# 27

# EFFECT OF LOCATION

Bhumi is the term for earth, or the land that we live on, in Ayurveda. Thus, both *Desha* (country or land) and *Jala* (water) are given importance in Swasthavritta and they are believed to have an effect on *Prakriti* (nature or constitution). Accordingly, regimes were developed to cope with the effects of one's location.

Land was broadly classified as –

1. *Jangala Desha* – areas of lush vegetation, but with an overabundance of Vata, requiring Vata alleviating foods and activity.

2. *Anupa Desha* – wetlands, with an overabundance of Kapha, requiring Kapha alleviating foods and activity.

3. *Sadharana Desha* – places which are normal in that the tridoshas are in equilibrium and people are hale and hearty.

*Vasasthana* is the term for residence and it was recommended that a residential place like a house should be constructed on the south-western side of a plot, which should be on high ground, in pleasant environs with plenty of fresh air and capable of nurturing trees and plants. Residences for the normal folk was proscribed, however, for locating in the vicinity of places such as the king's palace, temples, and from offensive locations such burial or cremating grounds, tanneries and factories. They were also told to avoid triangular grounds.

*Bhumi Shuddhi* is the term for the process of purifying or sterilising land to render it fit for residing. The process could involve a combination of washing, burning, vermicidal and germicidal treatment, such as Vidanga and Neem, and employing heating systems during the cold weather and cooling systems during the warm.

The *Paakshaala* or kitchen is to be constructed in *Agnimule* right side of east portion of the house precious for constructing a kitchen. This area must get clean and fresh air and plentiful light, which, in the modern day, may necessitate use of exhaust fans and appropriate lighting systems. The kitchen is to be located as far from the lavatory as possible.

For pastoral communities – and Ayurveda traces its roots to just such communities – cowsheds and stables were to be located as far from the actual residence as possible.

# SCHOOL HEALTH PROGRAMMES

The importance of Swasthavritta for schools may not be overstated. Not only are they centres for large populations and so prone to becoming centres for the spread of infection, but they are also places where the young congregate for learning by curricula as well as from example, and formative minds are likely to remember and practise what they have imbibed here for the rest of their lives.

Schools must be provided, therefore, with a good building, constructed in healthy and harmonious surrounds. Students must be provided with desks and proper equipment. Also necessary is that a medical examination should be conducted atleast once every year, if not more frequently. Such examination may be conducted by Ayurvedic practitioners as well. In addition to their studies, students must be provided with exposure to modern media – pamphlets, newswpapers, radio, television and audiovisual aids to learning. They should also be taught the basics such as the correct methods of brushing teeth, washing, bathing and principles of hygiene. Exercise, activity and even play is very important and facilities are required for this. They need to be coached in the use of community facilities such as lavatories which need to be segregated by gender. Today's children are the future citizens who will determine the direction of the country.

# FAMILY WELFARE PROGRAMMES

The purpose of family welfare programmes which are run by the state, is to generate well being in society at the level of individual families. As birth rates increase dramatically across many nations, the role of family planning becomes increasingly relevant throughout such countries of the world.

For enhancing the health of the family, the husband, the wife and their children, planned parenthood, of which antenatal and postnatal programmes are a part, need to be developed for the woman and her child. In India, such projects, which are called Maternity and Child Health Programmes, have been planned for implementation from the Public Health Unit (PHU) levels upwards to the level of major institutions. Ayurvedic systems of treatment have been duly recognised, and in order to provide the benefits of Ayurveda to the general public, each Public Health Centre is supposed to have at least one male and one female Ayurvedic doctor. There are a number of schemes at the national and the state levels, involving Ayurveda – unfortunately, most have not been properly implemented.

With the population increasing the way it is, appreciation of the necessity of family planning, which is a part of the broader issue of family welfare is laudable. However, a criticism that may be levelled with some justification is, that the policy on family planning should be one throughout the country, with no differentiation of caste or religion, without any attempts at appeasing any particular section of the populace. Also, there should be provisions for dealing with cases of sterility and greater attention to health measures aimed at mother and child.

As explained in some detail by the author in an earlier treatise, titled 'Family Planning in Ayurveda', the issue of family planning was recognised and addressed in India, much before it was in the rest of the world. Accordingly, mechanical systems of contraception, such as sheaths similar to the modern day condom, was used even in ancient days. Not only did it prevent contraception without the sort of side effects associated with a drug regime, it also prevented the spread of sexually transmitted diseases like AIDS and syphilis.

In modern India, it is also recognised that for controlling population incentives may be required to be given to the general populace. One such example is that of some states of the union which allows its employees special leave, followed with an extra increment in pay, for their **Vasectomy** operation, a simple procedure of cutting the vas deferens and re-tying the tubes after separation. While this applies to males, procedures applicable for the female can be Tubectomy – the 'female' equivalent of vasectomy, by fixing a loop (*lippis*) or by taking contraceptives – which can be either modern or Ayurvedic, and by use of spermicidal applications.

# 30

# PROPHYLACTIC MEASURES

Prophylaxis is the term that applies to prevention of disease before it can manifest. Prophylactic measures range from vaccination, which is conditioning the body to fight off infection, to use of covers or sheaths so that infection cannot reach vulnerable areas of the body. Modern day Ayurveda advocates the use of allopathic medicine for prophylaxis, as well as traditional prophylactics of Ayurveda.

Accordingly, vaccination, which is a relatively modern development, is recognised by practitioners of Ayurveda, as a must to be administered to children for its capability in preventing diseases such as smallpox, diptheria, whooping cough, tetanus, polio, typhoid, measles and some forms of pulmonary tuberculosis in later life. Vaccination for adults is also recognised as useful in the prevention of some forms of hepatitis and jaundice. The table given below outlines how some common vaccines should be administered.

**Tetanus – to be administered when the woman is pregnant**

16 – 20 weeks Tetanus Toxoid (first dose)

20 – 24 weeks Tetanus Toxoid (second dose)

36 – 38 weeks Tetanus Toxoid (third dose)

**For the infant**

| | | |
|---|---|---|
| 3 – 8 | months | Smallpox BCG<br>Triple antigen<br>Oral Vaccine |
| 8 – 12 | months | Measles |
| 18 – 24 | months | Triple antigen booster dose<br>Polio drops |
| 5 – 6 | years | Diptheria and Tetanus (at the time of admission to school) |
| 10 | years | Tetanus Toxoid<br>Typhoid |
| 16 | years | Tetanus Toxoid (before leaving school) |

There is a system of classification of disease in Ayurveda, based on the causative factor. Briefly, these are –

**A.** Epidemic diseases caused by imbibing contaminated food and drink
1. Antrik Jwara (internal fevers such as Typhoid)
2. Vishuchika (Gastroenteritis)
3. Atisara (Diarrhoea)

**B.** Airborne diseases
1. Masoorika (Measles)
2. Romantika
3. Yakshma (Tuberculosis)
4. Kapha Jwara

**C.** Diseases that spread through direct contact with it
1. Dhanusthambha
2. Jalasantarasa (Hydrophobia)
3. Upadamsha (Syphillis)

**D.** Diseases that spread through *Pipeelika* (a type of ants)
1. Antrik Jwara (internal fevers such as Typhoid)
2. Vishuchika (Gastroenteritis)
3. Atisara (Diarrhoea)

**E.** Matkuna Dwara
1. Kushta Roga (Leprosy)
2. Twak Roga (Skin disease)
3. Kaala Jwara

**F.** Kshudra Patanga Dwara
1. Granthika Jwara (Glandular fever)

**G.** Makshika Jwara – Vishama Jwara
1. Netrabhishyanda (Conjunctivitis)
2. Antrik Jwara (Enteric Fever)

**H.** Dhamsha Masaka Dwara
1. Vishama Jwara

**I.** Yuka Dwara
1. Aavrtika Jwara (Relapsing Fever)

In addition to medicinal cures and the use of medicated water, Ayurveda advocates the affected to employ procedures such as a change of place, Prayashchitta (penance), Mangala, Japa, Homa, Bali, Yagna, praying, invocation, showing respect for elders, for gurus and brahmins, donating to charities and exhibiting goodness.

*Ghoshana* is the term for an announcement in Ayurveda, and such an announcement to the concerned health authorities is mandatory when a death occurs due to an epidemic disease.

Extending this to the modern world, a proper announcement to the effect must appear in the media, whether radio, television or the newspapers. Patients suffering from epidemic disease should be isolated in hospices set aside for the purpose, in environs with good lighting and air. Utensils, clothes and personal effects of the person must be sterilised using proper reagents. Vermicides, vaccines and antibiotics may all be employed appropriately, as well as procedures such as burning, heat claving and fumigation. Some traditional substances known for their sterilisation and antibiotic properties are Neem leaves, Romaraji leaves, Tulsi, Karpura (camphor), Devadaru and Sarjarasa and can be used for Dhoopana (fumigation), and, as both dry and fluid chemicals. Nimba Patra (Neem leaves), sulphur, black Jeera, Dhoopa, Rala and Lobanes are known for their anti-pollution effects as well.

Sushrutha had developed a procedure for fumigation by preparing a compound of mustard, Neem leaves, salt and ghee, and fumigating daily for a period of ten days. This works equally well in modern times, and the properties of Neem in the form of lotions, drops and as liquid preparations are known worldwide. Human excreta from patients of typhoid, tuberculosis and measles requires to be collected in a vessel and either burnt or buried. Bacteriocides must be employed to cleanse the clothes of patients.

A dead body is called *Shava* and the Shavas should be either cremated, or, with some care, buried after cleansing with a disinfectant during an epidemic. Vectors such as flies and ticks should be rooted out employing insecticides.

Generally, good nutrition has an important role to play in building resistance in a person against infection and special food will help many from being effected. However, the quality of nutrition has no effect on some forms of epidemic disease, such as the plague, tuberculosis and AIDS.

## Some Contagious or Epidemic Diseases

*Kushta Roga* or Leprosy is caused by *Lapramatous lepra* and can spread through vectors such as flies and mosquitoes or even people. The prone happen to be those who are poor and those whose profession dictates a level of physical contact with the general public, such as beggars, washermen. barbers, cooks, clothes salesmen and prostitutes. Public facilities, such as public baths, may often be a source of the disease.

Malaria is spread through a vector, the Anopheles mosquito. Preventive measures against malaria employ the use of mosquito nets as well as mosquito repellants to keep the insect carrying the infection at bay. Medicine, allopathic and Ayurvedic may also be taken as prophylactic. These should be taken with the proper advise of an Ayurvedic doctor. Other measures to control the spread of malaria are to spray stagnant pools of water with a pesticide. The juice of Neem leaves is one such good agent which has a minimal side effect. Garbage from the kitchen should be buried in pits so as not to provide a food and breeding source for colonies of mosquitos. Fumigation inside the house, with Tulsi or Neem powder, is useful in controlling the mosquito menace. Those species of fish which eat mosquito larvae may also be released into ponds and lakes.

The Central Council of Ayurveda has developed an ague mixture of Arkashala into a tablet form, which goes by the name of Ayus-64. A Bangalore based company manufacturing ayurvedic preparations, called Maxpharma, has developed Malleril. Seeds of the plants called Karanja (*Pongamia Glabra*), Mahasudarshana Kashaya, the herbs Mrityunjayarasa and Jwarankusha, and camphor and garlic were some of the earlier forms of fighting off Malaria. Public education about malaria is a must and should employ all arms of the media.

The Plague is a contagion which has flared up repeatedly over the ages, in diverse and far flung communities. Called *Vatalika* or *Granthika Jwara* in the terminology of Ayurveda, it was recognised that plague is spread through rats mainly, although mosquitoes could also play a part in spreading contagion by feeding on infected rats and then passing on the infection to humans. Accumulation of garbage leads to a multiplication in the population of rats by providing them with both food and a habitat, and this, increases the likelihood of rat-borne contagion such as plague. Control of such epidemics requires control of the rat population, they need to be killed. It also requires controlling the mosquito vector through the methods outlined above, such as fumigation. Application of mustard and neem oils are useful preventives as was demonstrated during a recent outbreak in Gujarat.

Typhoid is known as *Antrika Jwara* in Ayurveda. From the earliest days, patients with symptoms of typhoid used to be removed to a hospital for treatment. A discovery made by Ayurveda was, that attacks of typhoid occurred with greater frequency during the cold season, that the virus spreads through airborne transmission, inflaming the throat and respiratory tract before affecting the other parts of the body. It is highly contagious and infects on contact with the infected person, and his or her faeces, urine, clothes and even utensils. During epidemics, public gatherings were proscribed and prophylaxis for the individual consisted of gargling with salt water to prevent kapha, and use of cleansing agents and disposal, generally by burning, of possibly infected material. Modern day Ayurveda recognises that useful vaccines have been developed to combat this menace.

Tuberculosis, caused by Bacillus tuberculosis, is known as *Shosha* or *Rajayakshama* in Ayurveda and is considered as predominantly a disease of the Kapha. Patients used to be removed to sanatoriums reserved for this purpose in the olden

113

days, but with the advent of oral chemotherapeutic agents, some level of control has been achieved. It is produced by –
1. Bacteria
2. Low bodily resistance
3. Breathing infected air
4. Obstructing natural urges
5. Physical exhaustion

The BCG vaccination is a preventive, but once a person has contracted the disease, it puts others at risk.This should be controlled by burning the patients sputum and use of antiseptics to kill the bacteria which patients release into their environment. The treatment is through a drug regime and there are a number of such in Ayurveda. Most importantly, treatment is by providing good nutrition, a diet rich in protein, such as milk, fish and eggs. Patients are advised to be careful about sexual indulgence.

Cholera, known as *Vishuchika* in Ayurvedic parlance, is caused by vibriocholera, a waterborne organism which contaminates rivers and wells. Unclean vegetables, milk and meals are the usual sources of this infection which causes acute vomiting and diarrhoea. The bodily excreta of the infected, their vomit, faeces and urine are highly contagious and flies and insects further spread the disease. Thus, disposal of excreta needs careful attention. Antiseptics such as chlorine must be employed to sterilise clothes, utensils and even household water. Food sold in public places must be proscribed, being a possible source of infection, and education and public awareness programmes should be conducted. Camphor has also been found to be quite an effective preventive agent. Red chillies and onions are beneficial as preventives in foods. The disposal of the dead should be preferably out of city limits, incineration being the best method of disposal.

Although now considered eradicated, Smallpox or *Masoorika* was a dreaded epidemic till recently. Caused by a virus, it was mainly protracted by children, spreading through droplet infection. Being highly infectious, patients were required to be kept in isolation. Treatment consists of the administration of septilin tablets for between one to two weeks. Earlier treatments were mostly palliative by nature while the disease ran its natural course and consisted of application of Neem or pepper paste externally and orally. Patients were put on diet, usually only milk.

Syphilis or *Upadamsha* is a sexually transmitted disease caused by the Treponema Palladeum organism which spreads through coitus. Typical symptom in an infected male is an ulcer on the penis. Improper treatment eventually leads to life-threatening situations, such as brain degeneration and cancer of the penis (*Sisnarbhuda*). Symptoms in females are far more covert but no less life-threatening. The disease can enter a dormant phase before flaring up later. In its secondary stage it often shows up as itchy rashes on the skin and as highly infective mucus patches in the mouth and with other infections such as condylomata. Thus it requires consultation with a doctor. Ayurvedic treatment consists of applications of Neem, Triphala decoction or mixed decoction of Guggulu and Triphala, at the rate of an ounce of decoction to a gram of Guggulu. Other Ayurvedic prescription involve Chopachini, Rasagandha, Kajjali, Brihatvangeswara, Suvarnarja Vangeswara, Saribadyarista, Sarbadi Ghrita and GT Ghritam, as per the advice of a doctor. The disease is very infectious, although transmission is prevented to an extent by employing sheaths and condoms. The disease can also spread through use of contaminated blood and needles. The disease is prevalent amongst prostitutes and so, frequenters of red light areas need to be sterilised.

Gonorrhoea or *Ushnameha* is another sexually transmitted disease and is caused by the organism Nesseria Gonorrhoea. The primary infection occurs in the genito-urinary tract, but the disease can then spread to the eyes, the anus (*Guda*), the bladder and the prostate, from the penis in the male and the labia majora in the female. Secondary infections, such as Trichomonas Vaginas can also result. A patient's utensils, clothes and dwelling place need to be sterilised with antiseptics. Qualified Ayurvedic practitioners use unguentum **(lepa)** – blood purifying medicines – for treatment. Some of these include MT Kashaya, MT Ghrita, GT Ghrita, Chandanasava, Chandanadi Vati, Rasamanikhya, Khadirarista and Saribadyarista.

# DISPOSAL OF FAECES

Excreta is very often a source of infection and a carrier of disease. Accordingly, its disposal, especially in temporary communities, is an area of major concern. Some basic methods of disposal are outlined below.

**Pail System:** A bucket is suitably placed for the man seated for defecation, so that all the faeces falls inside. After the act is completed, the bucket is removed and the waste centrally disposed. Some states in India, like Karnataka, have banned this system.

**Well Latrine:** A pit is dug and its upper surface covered with stone slabs with space for the faeces to drop through. When full, the pit is evacuated and cleaned. Typically, the pit may be as much as 20 feet wide and 10 feet deep.

**Bore-hole Latrine:** A hole, typically between 15 inches and 18 inches in circumference, is bored into the ground to a depth of 18 feet. This may be connected to a lavatory. The faeces drops into this bore.

**Permanent Latrine:** A permanent lavatory made for public use, is constructed between 15 and 100 feet from residences. The base of the lavatory is constructed on well-built, cemented platforms.

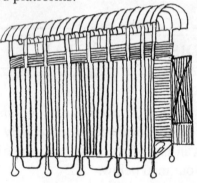

**Temporary Latrine:** For gatherings of a temporary nature, it is necessary to construct latrines. For this, a shed may be made using zinc sheets or similar material. The lavatories that are housed in this shed may employ any of the following alternatives – water closet, soil pipe, house drain or trap type. Faeces is collected in a cess-pool or pit and later dried and incinerated.

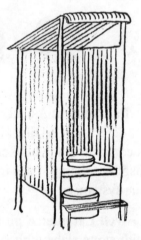

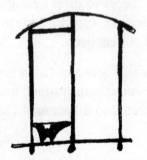

**Commode:** This is the 'Western' type of lavatory where the person defecating sits on a pot to pass motion. The pot is connected to the sewage or a cess-pit to which the faeces flows after flushing.

**Short Hopper:** This consists of a flush – a cistern of water being placed over the pot or the receptacle, into which the faeces drops. On pulling a lever or handle, a valve opens and the water rushes down through the force of gravity, thus flushing and cleaning the receptacle. Pipes leading from the bowl – as the receptacle is called – are connected to the central disposal system.

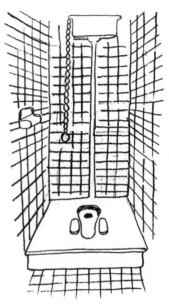

**Durable Faeces Disposal Way:** This has a long hopper in place of the short hopper system, which has been explained above. Otherwise, the principle is the same.

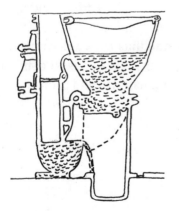

**Valve Closet:** Considered obsolete, the system operated with running water carrying away the discharge of faeces. It allowed for a place to keep the legs away from the stream of water.

**Traditional Method of Faeces Disposal:** It consisted of lavatories being connected to a sewage plant, where the refuse would be collected and separated from the water, which was the carrier. The water would be recycled, while the refuse would be turned into manure or compost.

From the early days of Ayurveda, certain occupations (*Vyavasaya*) were recognised as polluting and, thus, adversely affecting the health of the community. These were –

1. Rearing animals – including cows
2. Slaughter house operation – sheep, goat and pig being the more common ones
3. Treatment of dead animals – even such as incinerating their blood and organs
4. Skin tanning
5. Working in kilns, whether brick or lime

Extended to the modern day, this includes working in factories and manufacturing facilities of any of the following – paper, chemicals, cotton-gins, sugar, cement, silk, oil, rice and glass.

Such processing facilities emit noxious chemicals and gases, such as carbon dioxide ($CO_2$), carbon monoxide ($CO$), carbon disulphide ($CS_2$), hydrogen sulphide ($H_2S$), sulphur dioxide ($SO_2$), ammonia ($NH_3$), nitrous vapours, chlorine and halogenic compounds, and acids such as hydrochloric acid ($HCl$). This affects the skin, the lungs and respiratory system of the populace in their vicinity, and thus have a detrimental effect on the health of the community. Measures to contain the damage and the deposit of these harmful emissions must be given adequate attention.

# 32

# PUBLIC HEALTH ADMINISTRATION

In India, jurisdiction over the issues of governance are divided between the states that make up the union, and the centre, as the the national government is called. Health is a state subject, with individual states within the union determining what the policy should be for the citizens of that particular state. However, the Central Government, through its Health Ministry, tries to formulate a national framework for health issues through its National Health Policy, which takes cognisance of international thought on the subject, as projected by the WHO and the UNICEF. It sanctions grants to voluntary organisations, to NGOs as the non-governmental organisations are called, as well as to various wings of government services, such as the Central Government Health Services (C.G.H.S.) and health institutes, to implement central health policies. An elected member of parliament (M.P.) is appointed as the Central Health Minister to oversee the process.

Similarly, at the state level, an elected representative of the people, either a member of the legislative assembly (M.L.A.) or a member of the legislative council (M.L.C.) is appointed as the State Health Minister and controls and regulates the operation of the Health Department at the state level. To assist him in the discharge of his functions, he has a bureaucrat, usually designated as Health Commissioner or Health Secretary.

The commissioner, in turn, has his team of assistants who may be designated as Director, with attendant Joint, Additional,

Deputy and Assistant Directors. Typically, individual subject areas such as Malaria, Filaria, Leprosy, Tuberculosis and N.M.E.P. are allotted to a person of an Assistant Director's ranking. The states are composed of districts and each has its District Health Officer and District Surgeon. At the basic level, there are the Primary Health Centres (P.H.C) which are manned by Medical Officers who conduct prophylactic as well as curative programmes. Attached to these P.H.C.s are Junior and Senior Health Inspectors and A.N.M.S. and B.H.W.S. and Primary Health Units with doctors. In the state of Karnataka, the health and family welfare services provided by the government include programmes for family planning and eradication of smallpox and chickenpox.

A senior medical professional, drafted from the medical wing of the health services, is designated as Medical Director and regulates the activities of all medical colleges. These colleges provide training grounds for medical professionals and doctors such as A.N.M.S.s, opthalmologists and physiotherapists. There are nursing colleges also for training to paramedics and nursing staff.

Among the prominent international organisations which have assisted in health matters at the grassroot level and have assisted both state and central governments are the World Health Organisation (W.H.O.) and the United Nations International Children's Emergency Fund (U.N.I.C.E.F.). The WHO is headquartered in Geneva in Switzerland, and per declarations, such as the one at Alma Ata in 1978. It regulates the health of communities around the world. Delhi happens to be the headquarters of the WHO for South-east Asia. The UNICEF is a major branch of the United Nations Organisation (U.N.O.) and was created in 1946 to expressly cater to the needs of mother and child. Other prominent organisations to have contributed to the world community are the Red Cross (and Crescent) and the Rockefeller Foundation.

# 33

# AYURVEDA AND FAMILY PLANNING

The World is fast becoming grossly overpopulated as the human population alone approaches the 700 crore or 7 billion mark. Some 31% of this population is concentrated in South Asia, 21% in East Asia, while almost 12% populate Africa, 10% Europe, a little over 9% Latin America and just 6% populate North America. The population of India alone accounts for more than a billion, numbering about a 105 crores at the moment. These huge numbers are such, that there are just not enough resources to go around. In the next four hundred years or so, the world would have exhausted most of its non-replenishable energy producing minerals. The situation is much worse for a country like India, which is straining to provide even the basics to its citizens by way of food, clothing and housing.

It therefore becomes the bounden duty of every citizen, especially in an over-populated country like India, to contribute towards retarding and reversing this trend of growth in number of people. Otherwise, our society will degenerate into one of slums and shortages. Family planning is therefore a vital issue for modern society.

Family planning methods have been in vogue in a number of civilised societies from time immemorial, not just as a method of controlling population, but also because there are repeated and prolific childbirth endangers the health of the mother and endangers and impoverishes her children. Much attention has been given in Ayurveda on this issue and many ancient societies adopted family planning practices from Ayurveda.

**Developments in Ayurveda on Family Planning**

| | |
|---|---|
| BC: 1500 | Brihatagnya Kopanishat |
| BC: 1200 | Atharvaveda |
| BC: 1000 | Puranyuga |
| BC: 300 | Vatsayana Kama Sutra and Kousik Sutra |
| AD: 800 | Ratirahasya |
| AD: 1400 | Rasartana Samuchaya |
| AD: 1600 | Ananga Ranga, Bhava Prakasha and Brihat Yoga Tarangani |
| AD: 1800 | Ratimanjari and Yogaratna Samuchaya |
| AD: 1900 | Bhaishajya Ratnavali and Brihat Nighantu Ratnakara |

In the Kousik Sutra there is a vivid description of Vasectomy for the male and Tubectomy for the female.

One of the earliest texts, the Mahanarayanapanishad, deemed that Dharma was the greatest of all virtues. Dharma being belief in a code of conduct. In the Mahabharata it was stated that *"Dharmo Rakshati Rakshitaha"*, meaning, Dharma protects the person who practices it. Dharma changes with the times and Dharmas are relevant to the conditions of that epoch. Thus, though the Rigveda started by saying *"Dash ashyam Putran Adehi"* or allowing ten children for a couple, it later modified this allowance to *"Astaputra Soubhagya Vati Bhava"* - *"Puman To Jayam Puman Anujayatham"*, which means that eight children are a blessing. This was evidently on the premise, that there was a case for preventing and limiting the number of childbirths for any individual mother.

By the Subhashita period this had changed to *"Varameka Guni Putraha"* or, to limit progeny to just one, for, according to the Shatapata Brahmana, it was not possible to go to Heaven

124

without begetting a child. The wife was considered just one half of an individual and no divorce was allowed.

For most of that era, prostitution was forbidden and it was incumbent upon both man and wife to undergo Panchakarma therapy, as well as to ingest Rasayana and Vajeekarana drugs orally, along with milk of high quality, in order for their progeny to be potent, powerful and intelligent. Gradually though, it was left to the family itself to decide how many children there should be and if the size was already large the parents would practice measures to control pregnancy. These methods consisted of *Garbhasrava* and *Garbhapata* in accordance with the Kama Sutra, Bhava Prakash and Yogaratnakara. It was realised that both, not having a child, as well as, too many of them, were unnatural and potentially harmful states for any family. Though it was necessary to have children for happiness, in this and the other world, it was recognised that having too many, was a problem.

In ancient India, marriage was meant for propagating the race and for the continuity of the line through progeny, not mere sexual satisfaction. As survival rates after childbirth improved, the original edicts were modified accordingly. In fact Ayurvedic doctrines had postulated that unlimited growth of population results in *Matsya Nyaya*, with individuals resorting to cannibalistic behaviour, literally and metaphorically. This very sound principle should be considered relevant to our modern world and with over-population being as it is, it becomes incumbent on society to impose restrictions on family size.

The methods developed by Ayurveda to limit childbirth were:
1. *Brahmacharya* or celibacy
2. Avoiding coitus during *Rutukala*, the period when the woman is most fertile
3. Coitus during *Anrutukala*, the 'safe' period

125

4. Use of vaginal jellies, plugs and douches for contraception
5. Use of sheaths and such contraceptive aids for the male
6. Contraceptive preparations that would act on the semen and ovum
7. Aborteficients
8. Promoting social sanctions against promiscuity and encouraging the maintenance of the marriage bond
9. Surgery

**Terminology:** *Garbha* is the term for the process of conception. *Jeeva* or life (the foetus), forms with the union of *Shonita* (ovum or egg) and *Shukra* (sperms) and Garbha occurs only during the period in a woman's menstrual cycle known as Rutukala. Coitus during this period will produce Garbha provided that the Shonita, Sukra, and Garbhashaya (the uterus) are all healthy.

**Brahmacharya** or celibacy was commonly adopted by many to avoid conceiving further children. Brahmacharya meant the total avoidance of coitus.

**Rutukala** is the term for the period of twelve days in her menstrual cycle when a woman has ovulated and is at her most fertile. Avoiding coitus during this period will naturally decrease the risk of her becoming pregnant.

**Anurutukala** is the term for the days other than Rutukala during her menstrual cycle. Coitus during Anurutukala thus has a low risk of pregnancy unless the woman suffers from irregular menstrual cycles.

**Contraceptive Aids for the Female:**
These consist of applications of jellies and douches in the vagina, that have spermicidal properties and will kill sperm,

or, plugs to prevent entry of sperm. Some of the traditional techniques developed by Ayurveda are -

(a) Treating the vagina with a decoction made from the root of the *nimba* (Azadirachta Indica) plant.

(b) Lining the vagina with the powdered root of the *dhatoora* (Dhatoora Alba) plant.

(c) Applying inside the vagina, before intercourse, a cotton swab soaked in a mixture of castor and gingelly oils. Alternately the vagina may be swabbed with powdered rock salt dipped in til oil.

(d) Painting the vagina for seven days with the powdered seed of the *palasa* (Butea Frondosa) plant mixed in honey.

(e) Mixing the powders of jaggery, the seeds of the *Madanapala* plant (Randiadumetorum), the seeds of the *Drona* plant and *Yavakshara* can make a suppository. The mixture is then soaked in milk of Snuhi for a few hours and constitutes the suppository for the vagina.

(f) Application of pastes made from powdered *Bala, Languli, Bhunimbha, Devadali and Koshataki* roots, to the umbilicus of the woman.

(g) Irrigating the vaginal passages after coitus with a mixture of *Spatika* (Alum), *Jambeera Rasa* (lemon juice) and the water of rock salt.

Such applications are called Lepa.

## Some Contraceptive Aids for the Male:

Contraceptive aids for males consist of either spermicidal applications or sheaths such as condoms, which contain the ejaculate and so prevent the sperm from contact with any part of the vagina. *Mention of sheaths may be found in Vatsayana's Kama Sutra. Evidently, they were made of thin metal sheets of the thickness of a feather.* They could be of either the perforated kind or the un-perforated kinds. Shukrahara is the term used for spermicidal action and drugs with such action are:

1. **Twak Patra** or **Dalchini**
2. **Yavanika**
3. **Mishreya**

**Contraceptive drugs taken orally that work by affecting the semen and the ovum:**
These are based on Charaka's principles developed when he observed the etiology of delayed pregnancy in fertile women. He studied coitus during Anurutukala, the aggravation of Doshas in sperm and ovum, effects of dietary deficiency on ability to conceive and the gamut of activity involving sexual intercourse. That *Balasamakshaya* (debility) and *Manasika Abhitapa* (anxiety) affect and delay conception. Accordingly, Ayurvedic drugs were developed over time, notable among which are the ones described in the Kama Sutra, the Bhava Prakash and the Vaidyajeevana of the seventeenth century and the Yogarathnakara of the nineteenth. These recipes are touched upon below, but they should only be applied with advice from a proper Ayurvedic physician.

**Recipes for oral contraceptives from Bhava Prakash:**
(a) *Japakusum, puranaguda* (matured jaggery) and *aranala* (kanji) are taken in equal proportion to make up a dose of 5 tolas. One dose a day is taken for a week.
(b) Mixing 2 grams each of powdered Pippali (Piper Longum) prepare a daily dose, *tankana* (Borax) and *vidanga* (Embelia Ribes). This is taken for a week, immediately following menstruation.

**Recipes for oral contraceptives from Yogarathnakara:**
In his Streegarbhachikitsa chapter, Yogarathnakara described his formulations of oral contraceptives. These are:
(a) Kanji should be mixed with Japakusum and the mixture should be taken for three days after menstruation.

(b) 8 tolas of jaggery, which is at least three years old, should be taken every day for a period of fifteen days.

(c) A decoction should be prepared from *chitramool*, which is the root of the *Chitra* plant (Plumbaga Zeylanica) and drunk for the three days immediately following the menstrual period.

(d) Eating a quarter of the *Kadamba* fruit along with a drink of hot water will produce sterility in a woman.

(e) So will eating *Sarshapa* seed (Brassica Campherstris) along with drinking rice water.

(f) And so will eating the powdered seeds of the *Palasha* plant (Butea Frondosa) for three days.

(g) To prevent fertility, or conversely, to render a woman sterile for a period of two to three years, eating the pulp of just three castor seeds (Ricinuss Comunis) is enough.

**Other recipes for inducing sterility are:**

(a) Administrating *Swetagunga* at the rate of one on the fourth day of the menstrual cycle, two on the fifth and three on the sixth.

(b) A decoction prepared from the bark of the *Agnimanta* plant (Clerodendrum Serratum) to be taken along with rice water.

(c) Application of a paste made from the *Tanduliya* plant (Kirakusale Soppu) for three days.

(d) The root of the Snuhi plant (Euphorbia Nerufolia) is dried in the shade before burning and converting to ash. This ash is known as *Snuhi Bhasma* and must be taken for twenty-one days.

**Additional recipes for preventing conception are:**

(a) Administrating *Talisapatra* and *Gairitika* for three days.

(b) Tying the root of Dhatoora to the female waist during the period of Krishna Chaturdashi.

(c) Taking *Haridra* (Curcuma Longa) in water for six days after menstruation.

(d) *Katphaladi* (Myricaesulenta), *Shati* (Curucuma Zedoaria), *Nagakesara* (Mesuaferra), *Ajaji* (Cyminum Cynimum), *Haritaki* (Terminalia Chebula) and black *Jeera* (Carumcarvi) should be ground and mixed into pills of 1 tola, each which makes up the daily dose.

(e) The root of *Chitraka*, a total of fourteen black peppers (Piper Nigum), 3 tolas of Borax and 3 tolas of Haridra are mixed and ground to a fine powder. This is called the *Chitradkadi Choorna* and this should be taken twice every day in a suitable dose for eight days continuously.

**List of drugs with the capability of inducing sterility:**

1. Vidanga (Embelia Ribes)
2. Trapusa (Cucumis Satives)
3. Talisa (Abies Webbiana)
4. Snuhi (Euphorbia Nerifolia)
5. Shati (Curuma Zedoria)
6. Sarshapa (Brassica Campestris)
7. Palasha (Butea Frondosa)
8. Pippali (Piper Longum)
9. Maricha (Piper Nigrum)
10. Nagakesara (Myrica Esulenta)
11. Krishnajeeraka (Carum Carvi)
12. Champaka (Michelia Champaka)
13. Ajaji (Caminum Cynium)
14. Badara (Zisphus Jujuba)
15. Chitraka (Plumbaga Zeylanica)

**Abortificients** are those drugs, foods, chemicals or foods that bring about abortions and *Garbhapatana Vidhi* is the term for Methods of terminating pregnancy. Some of these methods are outlined below:

(a) Oral ingestion of three parts of the roots of *Dadima* (Punica Granatum) with one part of *Gunja*.

(b) Oral ingestion of 3 tolas of a paste made from *Nirgundi* (Vitex Negundo) mixed with Chitramoola and honey.

(c) Insertion of objects, such as the stem and leaves of *Eranda* into the vagina, effective until the fourth month of pregnancy.

(d) The stool of a horse ground into liquid *Kanji*, then filtered and mixed with rock salt and *Grasury Taila*.

Methods of family planning and population control extend beyond contraception or the termination of pregnancy. In some segments of society it is customary to marry young. Delaying the age at which couples marry is one method, reducing the number of times the woman is going to become pregnant. Not only do the number of children born to a mother come down, but, there are benefits for her overall health and physical condition.

## Current Developments in Family Planning

Having looked at some of the methods practiced in Ancient India, the bulk of which continue to be relevant and find applications today, it is time to touch upon aspects of family planning which are current.

## The Relevance of Ayurveda

When a comparison is made between Ayurveda and mainstream Medicine, it is evident that Ayurveda is relatively inexpensive. This applies to every aspect of cost, whether it is developing new medicine, drugs, and techniques of treatment or even in the actual treating. With very little capital expenditure on Research & Development to tap its potential, it is inevitable that Ayurveda will contribute affordable solutions to family planning and all of medicine. The lines of treatment and the drugs outlined above are surely worth further exploration.

## The Oral Ayurvedic Contraceptive Pill

A development worth a note, is the outcome of the research conducted by Dr. I. Sanjeeva Rao, Project Officer at the Central Ayurvedic Research Institute, Hyderabad, Andhra Pradesh. This is the contraceptive developed out of Ayurveda called *'Prikalpa'* which is available in the form of 500 mg. Tablets.

Most inexpensive, it is meant to be taken by women at a dose of twice a day for just five days. This dose prevents pregnancy for a period of around five years.

## Popular Methods of Avoiding Pregnancy

**For the Male,** this consists of mainly using the sheath or condom, which covers the male organ so that on ejaculation, the ejaculate stays within this sheath and none of it, touches, or is in contact with the female genitalia. Naturally this sheath should be free from holes or punctures. Generally made of polythene and its derivatives, or rubber derivatives, some of the popular brands are Durapac, from Durex in England, Gold Coins from Watch & Co., Japan and the indigenous Nirodh.

Coitus Interruptus or withdrawing the male organ from the genitalia when ejaculation is imminent is commonly employed.

**For the Female,** a number of methods are in vogue and these are outlined below:

1. **Diaphragm and Jelly** - Spermicidal jelly is applied to a diaphragm, which is then placed in the opening of the genitalia. The diaphragm blocks incoming sperm while the jelly with its destructive action provides an additional

safeguard. Diaphragms are available in sizes from 50 to 105 mm. in circumference with intervals of 2.5 to 5 mm. Size should be selected to ensure a proper fit.

2. **Lipp's Loop** - The loop is a wire instrument which is inserted into the vagina by an expert midwife (ANM) or a lady doctor, as is done with another similar instrument, the copper 'T'. Both prevent pregnancy. Usually, the slight initial discomfort wears off and these can be in place without requiring replacement for periods of five years. In rare cases, there are complications such as profuse bleeding.

3. **Chemical contraceptives** - formulated either as foam tablets, or, contabs of jelly and cream, they are to be applied before the act of coitus, after which, the genitalia must be washed thoroughly. Jelly may also be applied in the vagina by using a special syringe meant for the purpose. This syringe must be cleaned and disinfected thoroughly between uses. These applications are only moderately successful in averting pregnancy. The success rate of jellies, for instance, is only in the region of 60%.

   Durex Products, New York and Mumbai, manufacture a popular brand of foam tablet, Durafoam, while the British Drug House, London, manufactures a range of jellies. Such products are available at medical shops and at family welfare centres run by the Health & Family Welfare services.

4. **The Safe Period** - In any woman, only one ovum is released by her ovaries in a month, that is one ovum for one menstrual cycle. The ovum is motile and active for just 68 hours and the male sperm for just 48 hours. Sexual activity, during the ovum's 68 hour time window, presents the highest chance of pregnancy, with risk of pregnancy

declining progressively thereafter. Thus, if the lady partner menstruates on the first Monday of a month, the period when she runs the lowest, almost negligible, risk of pregnancy, or the 'safe period' for coitus is until the next Monday. However, the cycle of menstruation and its characteristics differ from person to person and from time to time. So, this method of preventing pregnancy has at best a 95% chance of being successful.

## Sterilisation

Once a couple have had children and do not want any more, sterilisation of either partner becomes an option for consideration. The procedure for sterilising the male partner is known as Vasectomy, while the procedure for sterilising the female partner is known as Salphingecetomy. Generally these are conducted by cutting and tying the tubes and tracts through which semen flows and most such procedures are reversible.

**Vasectomy** is a very simple surgical procedure nowadays, requiring barely fifteen to twenty minutes to conduct. With proper precautions of asepsis, it is generally quite safe with no later complication.

**Salphingecetomy** is more complicated in comparison and requires hospitalisation. An undertaking is required from the couple before it is conducted.

# PART B

# THE SCIENCE OF SOCIAL AND PERSONAL  HYGIENE

*(SAMAJIKA SWASTHAVRITTA VIJNANAM*
*AND*
*VAIYUKTIKA SWASTHVRITTA)*

# 34

# THE SCIENCE OF SOCIAL AND PERSONAL HYGIENE (JANAPADA DWAMSA)

An excessive congregation of too many people in one place will inevitably lead to epidemics of disease. These epidemics spread in two ways. The first way is when an individual is infected and becomes the host for the disease, in turn infecting others who come into contact or are in the carrier's proximity. The second way is when the disease is prevalent in the area and abruptly infects large numbers of people at the same time.

**Causes** – Ayurveda believes that man is composed of the Panchmahabhutas which are ever present in Nature. When these go wrong in Nature, they go wrong in the individuals, and this adversely affects health. Adharma or the lack of Dharma in any community is stated to be a cause for the vitiation of the elements, the water, air, and earth, and the time and place, which are the universally defining characteristics of any environment, just as sleep, hunger and the natural urges are the universally defining characteristics of all individuals. The age of the individual and the quality (or lack of) and the type of diet and food available, all have a bearing on epidemics taking hold.

It has been found that conducting certain processes of purification are beneficial during Greeshma (autumn), Varsha (monsoons) and Sisira Ritus. During the months of Shravana,

Karteeka and Chaitra Masa, the vitiation of Vata, Pitta and Kapha are to be restored. Often, a Dosha is only temporarily vitiated and may be easily cured by the simple treatments of *Langhana* (fasting) and *Paachana* (administering digestive stimulants). The *Samshodhana* Therapy, in particular *Jitaa Samshodhana Nairyetu Nateshan Punarudhbhavaha*, which has evolved over the millenia, is the one method of totally eradicating a disease.

A detailed treatise about Samshodhana Therapy titled *"Panchakarma Treatment of Ayurveda"* by the author, is available for those who may be interested in learning further.

In any case, Ayurveda has been postulating for six thousand years that a regulated lifestyle contributes to keeping the effects of epidemics and disease at bay. Thus food, drink, activity and setting limits on indulgence and obsessions are the key to a regulated life. Adequate sleep, some stimuli for the senses and control over promiscuity are necessary. Compassion, charity and shedding arrogance, all contribute to a mental state that helps ward off infections. All this is fortified by adopting a regime that includes Rasayana and Vrishya and acts such as cleaning teeth, attending to natural urges, exercise, Abhyanga, Snana (bathing) and Gandusha (gargling) and the like.

*Adharma* is the term for lack of regulation or wilful deviation towards the harmful. It may also be defined as the process of destroying one's health and life through harmful activity and food. Thus, sneezing and coughing on others and even yawning in an uncontrolled way can constitute adharma, as such acts spread infection. Ayurveda has proscribed, from the early days, eating food in hotels, brothels and choultries. Similarly, defecating and urinating in public places, like near a temple, in the village precincts, in tanks and public water reserves or on roads. It has advocated avoiding sources of infection such as dust and even exposure to bird droppings, as the individual thus affected not only suffers himself but can become a threat for the entire community.

Epidemics can also arise out of public facilities such as lavatories and any unclean place. Contamination of water by urine and faeces, whether animal or human in origin, is a major factor in the spread of diseases. Water is the essence of human life, being essential for drinking, cleaning, bathing and washing the individual and also for washing his surroundings, for construction, to douse fires and for any number of other applications.

It, thus, becomes the duty of health officials, who have the onus of maintaining public health, to regulate the proper supply of clean food and purified water. Pragnaparadha is the term for violation of this code of ethics. Corruption existed even in ancient times, and officials would neglect their duties and functions, thereby exposing communities to epidemics.

# 35

# COUNTRY OR AREA
# (DESHA)

Desha is the term for country or an area, and the characteristics of the area where a community is located often determines whether a particular epidemic could take hold in that community. Conversely, measures to eradicate disease have to take into account these area characteristics as well. This is a basic tenet of Ayurveda and so it is worth examining the thoughts of sages of yore, regarding the effects of location on health and their prescriptions.

They stated that residences should be built in square shapes, and if higher levels were proposed, these should be located towards the South and the East direction. Sounds which were considered harmonic, and thus beneficial, were the sound of elephants and horses, the flute, the veena and the ocean. It has since been established that sounds indeed have effects on health and sound waves have been used in medical treatments. As stated in the Mayamatha texts, and developed by the ancient Aryans nearly five thousand years ago, the flora of the location is useful for promoting health, and in fact can act as checks against epidemics. To name a few – *Nagakesara, Jati, Kamala, Gulabi, Patala, Gandhaka, Bilwa, Nirgundi* and *Ela*. On the other hand, deposits of bone, alkaline matter and marshes were known to be detrimental to health and to be promoters of epidemics. In the Griha Bhushana texts, it was opined that all things which are pleasing to the eyes and the senses, such as sunlight, breeze, fresh air, rain and foliage safeguard against disease. Obviously, despoiled locations spread pollution into the surrounding atmosphere and water, and promote and harbour bacteria. Such places require purification of Desha, a process of cleaning and removing obstacles to allow sunlight, fresh air and the like to come in. Simple but effective clean-up measures since early times were to allow cattle to graze on the lands, as cow dung and urine do have antiseptic properties. In fact, Maharajas used to drink diluted forms of cow's urine as a part of their health regime at some point of time or the other. Even today, the urine of a black cow is used by some sects of Brahmins during Upanayana. Current practise is to use chemicals as antiseptic for purification.

**Classification of Deshas:** The three broad classes of Deshas are –

1. Jangala Desha
2. Anupa Desha
3. Sadharana Desha

The Jangala Desha is characterised as a flat land with little foliage, strong winds and excessive sunlight. People living in such areas will be prone to problems of the Vata.

Anupa Desha is the exact opposite. Marshy, with excessive foliage and insufficient sunlight. Such areas are naturally more bacteria producing and people living in such areas will be prone to problems of the Kapha. Some typical manifestations of disorders of the Kapha being fevers, *Slipada* (Elephantiasis) and *Gulmas* (Fantom Tumour).

Sadharana Desha is the one where all the Doshas are balanced.

**Some Guidelines for Constructing a Residence** – While humans require housing for shelter, they have developed to a stage where their residences are more than mere shelters – a place for living, eating, catering to natural urges with privacy and a variety of activity. Accordingly, residences may be constructed with a number of rooms such as bedrooms, bathrooms, a study, guest rooms, kitchen, dining hall, storage and out-house facilities such as a cattle shed. Doors and windows must be provided, not just for connectivity but for ventilation and visual stimulation. The front of the house should have space and the surrounds should not have pools of stagnant or dirty water or drains, which may be the cause of offensive smells or collection of garbage and excreta. The house itself should occupy the high ground on the property, which must be cleared of rodents, snakes and other pests.

**Laying Out a Village** – In India, it is customary to constitute a council of five elders, called a Gram Panchayat, to oversee administrative matters of all villages, whether large or small. Although the constituent members may not be experts on the subject of health, it rests upon them to mobilise sections of villagers to ensure that the village precincts are kept clean. They must also interact with the concerned civic bodies to ensure proper supply of pure water. In the past, this often meant that they supervised the construction of wells, often within gardens of the village. Village dwellings should be fumigated with aromatic compounds to eradicate mosquitoes and other pests. The graveyard and cremation grounds should be located away from the residential part of the village and properly maintained. The village should have common facilities for the convenience of the community, at the very least, urinals and lavatory with a constituted body to clean these to keep them from becoming foul.

**Laying Out a City** – It is to be realised that the population of a city and its density is huge when compared with a village. It is important for cities to have wide roads and a cushion for expansion. The roads should be constructed with footpaths for the convenience of strollers. Cities should be positioned on higher ground than the surrounding countryside as this will help with the drainage. The city needs to set a minimum standard for all housing that may be built in it and these standards must prescribe a minimum area for an abode so that homes do not want for basic facilities. A basic minimum may be a kitchen, a bathroom with toilet, a bedroom, a dining space with, perhaps, provision for a puja room and a study. Attention is required for industrial areas and location of factories as these provide employment in addition to offering goods for consumption. Similarly, attention needs to be given to public places including centres of entertainment and recreation, such as sports fields, stadia and cinema halls. It is the duty of constituted health authorities, who may be either the municipality or corporation to inspect all locations to ensure adherence to standards. Per the tenets of Ayurveda, provision must be made for grazing spaces for animals and for gardens. A proper and adequate system for drainage is vital and this should provide for the growth in population over time. It is also vital to supervise effluent discharge by factories and industrial units as this sector is often the largest source of pollution. Waste disposal is a matter of much concern, and measures can include either digging deep shafts to receive waste, or landfills or sewage plants where a number of methods such as drying and composting or chemical treatment may be employed. Planting trees is good for all cities because trees remove noxious vapours from the air and replenish the atmosphere with oxygen. Playgrounds for the young are necessary and the city must provide for emergency services.

**An Educational Institution** – Educational institutions are the places where we nurture the citizens of the future and so they should be located on the best land available. Land of good quality, away from squalor and noisy environs. The building itself should be airy or properly ventilated and such as to allow plenty of light. Rooms should be large, at least a hundred and fifty square feet in area, with high ceilings of between nine and fifteen feet. It is worth noting that even the best institutes, by way of the advanced equipment they posses, often lose sight of providing basic amenities like enough chairs or washrooms and urinals, and in terms of cleanliness or maintenance. We advocate that schools and the like should provide students with meals during their study day.

# 36

# THE FOOD WE EAT
# (AHARA)

In the Kashyapa Samhita it is stated that *"Arogyam Bhojana Dheenam"*, which, loosely translated, means that people with proper eating habits will generally not require medicines. The foods that we eat supply combinations of Panchmahabhutas, the very stuff of nature and humans. In addition to the nutrient content of the food that we eat, however, the ancient thinkers had postulated that how we eat, an eating etiquette as it were, has a bearing on how effectively we use those nutrients. It was also postulated that the purity of the food eaten correlated with the purity of mind of the eater. Some of the guidelines on eating etiquette included – one should not allow any distractions to divert oneself while eating food; it is important that the mind stays focused on the meal. The meal should be eaten at a regular pace and food carefully chewed, neither too fast nor very slowly. It is important to wash one's face, mouth and hands before and after a meal. Food should be eaten in a congenial atmosphere, perhaps with friends, parents or relatives. The mood is important and food should not be eaten in a pre-occupied manner or too quickly, as this interferes with the secretion and the effectiveness of digestive enzymes. Eating food while sitting in a padmasana style helps the functioning of the Samana and Apana Vayus and so this posture is beneficial for digestion. The place where the meal is being eaten must have proper illumination, whether natural or artificial. An offering should be made before one's meal to either the poor or to animals. Food should be taken when one is hungry, within limits, taking care not to overeat. The food should be tasty and stimulating. It is important to enjoy one's meal.

On another level, it is important that previous meals have been thoroughly digested before embarking on the next, and also only after ensuring that natural urges such as excreting have been satisfied and the doshas are functioning properly. A signal that these are in order and that one's Samana and Apana Doshas are functioning properly is when the body feels light and active as opposed to feelings of heaviness in the body. Generally, the spacing between meals should be of approximately two *Yamas* or six hours duration, each Yama being three hours. Bhavaprakash was an authority on this issue and he stated that an interval of just one Yama between meals created a condition termed as *Rasavastha*, obstruction in the digestive passages leading to overproduction of Rasa, leading to *Ama* and allied conditions. Going beyond two Yamas without food results in loss of energy. It increases one's Dhatvagni and may reduce strength drastically.

The suitability of actual diet that is taken depends on a number of factors. These are – location, time of day, individual habit, whether the diet itself is beneficial or not and the climate and season. The amount of food that is suitable to eat, naturally, varies from person to person, depending upon individual constitution, the size of the eater and individual digestive powers, which should be sufficient to digest one's meal properly. Depending upon fat and other constituents, food which strains digestive powers may be termed as heavy. Heavy food should be eaten in half the quantity as "light" food. It is also important to balance solid foods with liquid. Solids should be ingested to the capacity of approximately half of one's stomach, while liquids should fill a quarter, leaving the last quarter free for the doshas to act upon the food. The meal should be composed of *Shadrasas* or six different tastes and include the Prithvi and Apbhutas. Its constituents should be a blend of the Snigdha or oily, the Ushna or hot, the Laghu or light and the Dravam or liquid. All food should be homologous with one's body. It should be pleasing to one's senses and the motor organs in colour, texture and taste. The ideal meal, according to Chanakya, consisted of red rice matured to sixty days after harvest, Mudga, salt, Amalaki, the Java type of wheat, pure water, ghee, honey and the flesh of Jangala animals. For vegetarians, he recommended a meal of milk and curd, ghee, Masha, Chanaka, Surama and vegetables, seasoned in butter or ghee. Modern day Nutrition would consider this as a total and balanced meal. The rice provides starch and carbohydrates besides some vitamins; the Mudga, wheat, meat and Masha the protein and minerals; the milk, butter and ghee, the fats, and honey and Amalaki, the additional vitamin and micro-nutrients.

Food, when eaten in the manner prescribed above, will in itself act as a preventer of disease because of the steady and balanced nutrition it provides the body on being properly digested. The Sara in the body will produce just the right amount of Rasa to extract the most from the nutrients, while forming adequate cellulose for Kitta – the functions of excretion of waste.

Some food substances which are taboo in Ayurveda are – the stale and those with any hint of putrification, those associated with stones, grass and hair, food which is reheated, which produces aversion and any which is very cold or insuffiently boiled or overcooked and heavily fried. Plants, vegetables and herbs grown on the roadside or in marshy places are also taboo. All the above are considered to be poisons for the body.

While detailed recommendations have been given by Charaka in the 27th Chapter and 344th Sloka of his treatise, the *Sutrasthana*, on the preparation of meals, some of the basics are, that ingredients must be mixed properly, and where they are to be boiled, the process should be thorough. Boiled milk digests far better than fresh. Saktu seasoned with Samskara, if fried, is difficult to digest – from which one gleans that fried and heavily seasoned food is difficult to digest. That butter-milk, which is a form of curd or yoghurt diluted with pure water, has excellent digestive properties. Besides providing nutrition in itself, it assists digestion and benefits complications of Kapha. It is the diet of choice when a patient is suffering from loose motions, abdominal pain, problem with piles, urticaria (*Sheeta Pitta*) or the sprue syndrome (*Grahani*).

Any meal that we eat is composed of individual items of food. While combinations of these items of food may often be synergistic, this is not always the case. Sometimes, combinations do not harmonise inside the body when ingested together and can create problems for digestion or other side effects and allergic reactions. Such combinations then become poisons for the body. For instance, equal proportions or even near equal proportions, of ghee and honey create adverse reactions in the body. So too does a combination of milk with meats and especially so when heated, definitely producing symptoms of indigestion. When dicotyledons are boiled with either rice or Khanji, as is often done while preparing a desert called Payasam, the combination will cause digestive problems in spite of each of the constituents being easily digested foods individually.

**Viruddha Ahara (Incompatible or Allergy Creating food):**
Dating back to Charaka's times, Ayurveda has explored the subject of foods that are antagonistic to the body and that can provoke allergic reactions. In Sloka 89 of Chapter 26 of his treatise, Charaka vividly describes the gamut of incompatibility of food. Broadly, eleven classifications can be made for such incompatibility, and these are –

1. **Deshaviruddha** – Foods which are unsuitable because they are the wrong ones for a particular location. These foods may be quite nutritional in another place.
2. **Kalaviruddha** – Foods that are unsuitable for climatic and seasonal reasons.
3. **Agniviruddha** – Foods that go against the Manda, Teekshana and Vishamagni.
4. **Satmyaviruddha** – Foods that do not suit one personally, or foods that are not homologous with oneself. Such foods may cause an allergy in one person but not the next.
5. **Aniladiviruddha** – Foods that cause imbalances of the Vata, Pitta and Kapha.
6. **Veeryaviruddha** – A mixture of foods that differ in potency or differ in property, such as mixing Ushna (hot foods) with Sheetha (cold foods). An example – combining a stimulant with a sedative.
7. **Kosthaviruddha** – Foods that strain or injure the digestive system of the body, the Manda, Madhya and the Krura Kostha.
8. **Avasthaviruddha** – Foods that are unsuitable because of one's personal condition at the moment, such as when one is fatigued or suffering from indigestion. These foods may be quite ingestible at other times.

9. **Vipakaviruddha** – Foods that are not taken in their proper sequence. For example, pungent substances (*Katu Vipaka*) if imbibed at the beginning of a meal may irritate the stomach. These may be ingested with no ill effects later in the meal once the stomach has been lined with gentler foods (*Madhura Vipaka*). Some Indian sweatmeats are meant for this purpose and fill the role of starters.

10. **Pramanaviruddha** – Food which may otherwise have no adverse effects when ingested in suitable quantity.

11. **Swabhava Viruddha** – Foods that do not suit one's nature or are antagonistic to one's natural instincts.

According to both Charaka and Vagbhata, as stated in Sloka 84 Chapter 26 of the *Charaka Sutra* and in Sloka 45 Chapter 29 of the seventh *Astanga Sutra,* these eleven kinds of food produce vitiation of the Rakta and act as poison. Thus, they are to be strictly avoided.

Impotency, erysipelas, ascites, *Vispota* (blisters), Unmada (insanity), Grahani or the sprue syndorme, Murcha, Mada, anal fistula, consumptive diseases, haemorrhagic disorders, neck disease, disorders of the nose and generative organs besides fevers can all result from eating incompatible food.

**Treating the Result of Eating Incompatible Food:** Levels of incompatibility of such food vary from person to person, depending upon individual constitution and habits. Factors such as whether one is in prime fitness, or exercising regularly, one's age, strength of digestive powers or has become used to and has at least limited immunity to, all play their part in the extent of reaction to incompatible food. Often limited quantities of such food, when eaten, produce no ill-effects although sustained ingestion is bound to produce any of the conditions listed above. Knowledge and awareness about such foods and using such information may be considered the first step in guarding oneself against illness. Once symptoms show up, taking emetics and purgatives and substances of the type that act in a way opposite to the action of the problem food, is another. Naturally, a change in diet is called for. Sometimes incompatible food items are quite addictive and require a process of weaning away from. One method is to introduce suitable food to the extent of a quarter of one's intake in stages till finally eliminating the noxious from one's diet. For more acute conditions, liquid food, in the form of *Peya,* and fluids is usually given, and soups, gruels, butter-milk and milk are suitable ways. Such potions are called *Yavagu.* Other foods with similar function are *Manda*, Peya and *Vilepi.* Manda is the term for clear soups. By adding small amounts of rice, the resulting gruel is called Peya. The term for a thicker broth is Vilepi, and Vayagu is the thickest of all. Together, the four form a part of Dravas or meals in liquid form, and are meant to be taken at the conclusion of meals. Like milk, they provide nutrition besides soothing internal organs. Butter-milk helps with both digestion and assimilation of food and also aids all the processes of excretion of the body. Rava from wheat and dicotyledons can all be used in the stock for the additional nutrition that they lend. Drugs and other medication can be safely mixed with these for preparing curative potions, but the dosage should be appropriate to the particular base, whether Manda or Peya or other. Manda, being the thinnest, is also the lightest in terms of strain on digestion, while the others are progressively heavier and choosing between them is a matter governed by the state of the patient. The dosage of medication mixed should match this. Even healthy people find that preparations of Peya improves their feeling of well being.

# 37

# WATER
# (UDAKA)

All living beings require water to sustain life. Besides carrying nutrition from which all tissue matter and organs derive the energy essential for functioning, the bulk of all living cells is composed mostly of water. For humankind, the availability of pure or uncontaminated water has always been a vital issue. Sources of contamination are many, whether bacteria and germs or by way of excreta of animal life or because of rotting vegetation, notwithstanding artificial or man-made pollution of modern days. Thus, much of stored water is unfit for human use, unfit for not just drinking, but also for washing, bathing and even cleaning. In the *Astanga Samgraha,* it was said that the characteristics displayed by impure water include appearing thick, foamy, without taste or offensive, if it causes sensations of burning or heat without being actually heated, or if it is teeth-chilling cold. Such water is deemed unfit for human use.

Ayurveda recognised that the cause of many diseases is water borne and so advocated water harvesting. Collecting and properly storing rainwater and digging wells at distances from human habitat, so, distanced from polluting sources. Though sunlight has cleansing properties, as does running water to an extent, even rivers and channels have every likelihood of becoming contaminated through stagnating deposits of vegetative, animal or man-made matter. As the *Sutrasthana* states, water of the kind that displays the properties listed above will be spurned by bird and beast and will lead to disease – swelling of the body, anaemia, skin diseases, indigestion, dsypnoea, cough, rhinorrhoea, colds and tumours. Furthermore, contaminated water can cause heaviness in the body, fever, itching and rashes, abnormal thirst, enlargement of the glands (*Gandamala*) and typhoid.

**Pure and Impure Water – (Charaka:)** Pure water will taste slightly astringent and sweet and feel light and dry (quickly evaporating) to the touch. It will have no smell and, on drinking, will satisfy thirst immediately, altogether pleasurable to drink. It will relieve fatigue, cool the brain and invigorate the body. It will bring relief from feelings of Murcha, itching and burning to those suffering from these. Vitiated water will distend the belly, besides producing the conditions mentioned earlier.

Three types of water contamination –

1. *Plavita Mala* – floating contamination

2. *Gulita Mala* – dissolved contamination

3. *Vishajantu* – presence of germs and bacteria in the water Common sources of contamination include decaying matter such as dead bodies, when bacteria multiplies during the decaying process and trickles into water, sewage water and the seepage of sewage into soil. Khanija (metals) seeping into water supply is a common cause for the Gulita Mala type of contamination.

**Sushrutha's Methods of Water Purification**
*Marjana* and *Prasadana* were two methods employed by Sushrutha for purifying contaminated water.

Marjana is the term for water treatment when either heat or radiation is employed for cleansing it. Methods employed during Sushrutha's era were boiling water, or heating it by inserting bricks or iron pieces at very high temperatures and exposure to sunlight. It is now well-known that the ultra-violet radiation in sunlight has bactericidal properties.

**Prasadana** is the term for treating water with substances. Traditionally, Gomedaka Mani, Kathaka seed and Shaivala were employed. Present practice employs chemicals, bleaching powder for one, and later developments of many powerful chemicals with fewer side effects.

**Removing Plavitamala** – Simple methods of removing floating or suspended particulate contamination can be to just allow the water to settle for a period of time or to pass water through a fine sieve, such as a muslin cloth, when relatively limited quantities are required for use. When the storage method is being employed, powdered seed of Kathaka or Alum or a combination may be added to the water as these hasten the process of sedimentation. The water can then be filtered and supplied. Another method employed was to allow water to fall from great heights. This allows exposure to atmosphere, thereby oxidising bacteria to an extent.

Yet another method is known as the Three Pot Method – called respectively *Trustakea*, *Dandatraya* and *Udakamanchika,* which are placed on top of each other. The upper two pots have holes centred in their bottom, measuring between two and two and a half inches across. The hole in the upper pot is covered with grass, while the hole in the next pot is covered with a webbing containing charcoal. Water is then poured into the uppermost pot and it filters through to the bottom most one. By then, it is relatively pure.

**Removing Gulitamala** – A method of removing dissolved matter or improving the quality of offensive smelling water was, and is, to pour the water into a vessel of either gold or silver as these higher metals do not leach. To this water are added the flowers of lotus, *Nagakesara* and *Sampige*. This causes dissolved matter to particulate out and form a scum, which can then be removed by the other ways, already detailed. The heated water is then stored in a pot which is painted with lime.

**Removing Vishajantu** – Boiling is an effective method that kills most common forms of bacteria in water; and after boiling, the water can be filtered and the three pot method employed for further purification. Bactericidal drugs may also be used. Storage of water in copper vessels is useful as copper has anti-bacterial, anti-microbial, as well as anti-fungal properties.

By employing these and similar methods pure water was supplied to fairly large numbers of people in the towns that existed five thousand and more years ago.

*Anupana* is the term used for an antidote when the food that we eat lacks any one of the Shadrasas. When a meal consists of purely solid matter, for instance, the meal loses much of its flavour, besides producing indigestion. Water is Anupana for such a meal. Similarly, when a meal is mostly *amla* (sour) in composition, something sweet needs to be eaten to get rid of the resulting offensive smell in one's mouth. Refreshing beverages are also Anupana.

Sloka 419 of Chapter 46 of Sushrutha's work deals with this subject. In general though, both hot and cold water, Asavarista, Madya or alcohol, Yusa, Peya, fruit drinks and Dhanyamla are types of Anupana. Meats, milk and sour tidbits such as chooran and pickles can also function as Anupana, depending on personal tastes and the season. Quoting from Charaka's Sloka 326 of Chapter 27, bland foods must be taken for Pitta disorders while dry and hot foods must be taken for

Kapha disorders and soups prepared from meat stocks are good for weak and emaciated people. Cold water is the Anupana for wheat, curd, Madya and honey and even for cases of poisoning. In case of starchy foods, it is warm water. Sloka 47 in Chapter 8 of the *Astanga Sutra* prescribes butter-milk or the fluid from curds as the Anupana for dicotyledons, Mudga and vegetables.

Enough cannot be said about the benefits of pure water. It is good for the heart and blood circulation, it is cooling, it satisfies the body and also contributes to the intellect. Reference can be found in Sushrutha Sutra in Sloka 420 of Chapter 46. Water from Jangaldeshas is abundant in Vata, while water from Anupadesha is abundant in Kapha. The best natural water is called *Gangambu* and to be found as rain-water in airy places, with plentiful sunlight, in clean environs away from contamination.

**The Six Doshas of Vitiated Water** – Rainwater which falls through an unpolluted atmosphere has no morbid material in it and none of the Doshas are vitiated. It has all the positive qualities enumerated. With the effects of pollution and away from nature's cleansing agents, the sun, moon and air, it will develop smells, colour and tastes. Such water is vitiated and the types of vitiation are six. These are –

1. *Sparsha Dosha* or vitiation by touch. When water feels rough, invicid, burns or irritates irritation or causes of the teeth.

2. *Roopa Dosha* or vitiation of texture. When it has sediments or suspended matter such as mud, sand or plankton.

3. *Rasa Dosha* or vitiation of taste. When it has a bad taste.

4. *Gandha Dosha* or vitiation of smell. When it smells.

5. *Veerya Dosha* or vitiation of its properties. It produces symptoms and reactions in the drinker – pain in the abdomen, thirst, heaviness or excessive salivation.

6. *Paka Dosha* or vitiation of its digestive capability. Drinking it produces indigestion and constipation.

Vitiated water requires to be purified before it becomes fit for drinking purposes and methods of purification have been discussed earlier in this chapter. Additional measures for improving quality are adding Naga, Patala and lotus flowers for fragrance. Preserving potable water in pots of gold or silver or copper, or failing this, at least in pots of earthenware. *Gomedaka* roots and *Spatikamini* are effective dispersing agents.

**Traditional Methods of Storing Drinking Water** – The vessel containing the water is covered with a Phalaka and placed upon a tripod constructed from three eight-cornered cans. The vessel rests on a bed of grass of the Munja variety. Alternately, the vessel would be attached to a rope and suspended.

Lacking refrigerators, there were seven methods employed to cool drinking water –

1. Storing water in a wide mouthed vessel which allowed exposure to air
2. By keeing the vessel of water over another vessel containing already cold water
3. Stirring the water with canes
4. Storing water in a wide-mouthed vessel and fanning it
5. Pouring the water slowly through a coarse cloth
6. Packing the vessel containing water in cold sand
7. Hanging the vessel and swinging it through air

**River Water** – River waters were as important a source of potable water for the populace then as now. However, the ancients believed that rivers flowing westward provided water which was pure and light and good for use. Rivers that flowed southward provided water which was satisfactory, but water from rivers flowing eastward was 'not good' and treated with suspicion. This, quite naturally, derived from the topography of the area in the South-west region of India. It was also believed that water from Himalayan rivers was dangerous and could cause skin diseases, leprosy and anaemia, besides heart disease, oedema, headaches, elephantiasis and goitre, and that water flowing down the Mahendra Parvat produced elephantiasis, and affected the stomach.

They recognised, as modern science knows for a fact, that flowing water has properties of self-purification and the faster the flow the better the quality of water. Thus, rivers that flowed slowly gave water that took time to digest. They believed that though desert water was bitter and salty, it provided strength to the body, perhaps on account of the additional minerals such water contains.

Cold water was used for treating physical conditions. For people in a coma, those with bilious disorders, for relief when the weather was hot, for flushing poisons from the body, for treating alcoholics and a number of afflictions like burns, giddiness, bronchial asthma, fatigue and bleeding from the nose and mouth. Cold water for such purposes would first be boiled and then cooled.

Use of cold water was proscribed in case of chest pains, rhinorrhoea and sinusitis, nervous disorders, lockjaw, distension of the stomach, indigestion, fever, hiccups and for the administration of emetics and purgatives. Cold water was never drunk when eating ghee and oily substances.

Hot water was used for treating Vatadoshas and Amadoshas, as an aid to speedier digestion and to remove deposits of phlegm and fat.

# 38

# AIR POLLUTION

Air Pollution, which, in modern times, is an ever-present threat, has existed from the earliest civilisations. Fumes and poisonous gases were known to occur in concentration and signaled their presence by killing birds and worms. Such cases of pollution have been recorded by both Sushrutha and Charaka, and sometimes would be severe enough to cause an outbreak of colds and headaches, as well as episodes of monoplegia, hemiplegia, paraplegia and eye disease among the human populace. Severe pollution causing the death of animals resulted in carcasses being strewn across the countryside, resulting in a cycle of further pollution of the ground and the air, leading to epidemics and the prevalence of disease. Coping with the problem of pollution was a concern even in Sushrutha's days and, accordingly, he wrote his second Kalpasthana Chapters to address the subject.

**The portents of air pollution:** Abnormal atmospheric airflow creates conditions that are ripe for air pollution to occur, it being considered that presence of a slight breeze is the normal condition of our atmosphere. However, when air is stagnant it will not dissipate fumes and gases that is an inevitable byproduct of conglomeration of people. Again, when the wind blows from the wrong direction, it will carry with it pollution from sources such as tanneries and factories to places of habitat. This may take many forms, sometimes simply noise pollution and at others an offensive smell will be the signal for pollution. The severity of pollution is directly linked to the seasons because of seasonal wind patterns. Much severe pollution is insidious and may catch the community unawares at first, and it is only when disease occurs in the populace that cognizance sinks in. At the lower end of the scale, the symptoms take the form of headaches, breathing difficulty, giddiness and nausea. At the other end, it is capable of producing a variety of fevers and malaise, it can transmit epidemic disease such as smallpox (*Masoorika*), tuberculosis, gastroenteritis *(Vishuchika)* and cause people to become consumptive, and cause deformation of the foetus. Air pollution vitiates Pranavayu and sustained presence of pollution destroys contentment, saps strength and the very life force of people, reducing their life-spans, affecting their sensory and motor organs and resulting in abnormal behaviour.

**Purification of air,** as advocated in the second chapter of the *Kalpasthana* laid emphasis of removal and disposal of dead bodies, followed by the application of antiseptics. This took the form of burning of powders with antiseptic and sterilising properties and powders of *Laksha, Haridra, Athivisha, Abhaya, Aranala, Valka, Panchvalkala, Brahmi, Bhakuchi, Devadaru, white Sharshapa, Karnanja, Rala, Agaru* and even sulphur were poured on fires lit for the purpose, producing fumes for destroying bacteria and germs. Practise of Pranayama was then conducted as it regulates the Vata. That plants and sunlight are natural cleansing agents was recognised and encouraged.

It is believed that certain sounds have a beneficial effect on humans. Sounds made by horses, elephants and the playing of the flute are some. Thus, producing these sounds is a step towards safeguarding health. Residences should be located on high ground on the westerly side of any area and drugs like *Nagakesara, Jathi, Kamala, Gulabi, Dhanyakha, Patola, Gandhaka, Nimbha, Bilva, Nirgundi* and *Ela* should be burnt in the surrounds to overcome the effects of pollution. References from the *Mayamatha* book and the *Guda Bhushama* texts assert that epidemics rarely take hold in areas of great natural beauty and communities that enjoy happiness of mind and body. Also, when there is a normal amount of rain, breeze, sunlight and fresh air, such as they occur in Sadharana Deshas, epidemics are rare. Because the conditions of Anupa Desha with its excessive wetness and Jangala Deshas with its excessive dryness are peculiar, these areas are relatively prone to pollution related epidemics. A technique to clean polluted fields was to allow cattle to graze on them, their dung having antiseptic properties.

**Effects of Wind Direction**
**From the North** – when the wind blows from the North, it is believed by the pundits of South India, that it is a benign wind, sweet and not astringent in character, although cold, and will not vitiate the Doshas. It is good for people suffering from tuberculosis and poisoning.

Wind from the North though sweet, will also be salty and act against blood and Pitta. It will be bad for those suffering from diseases involving respiration. It will be dangerous for those with disorders of the Kapha and will sap the strength and affect the bodily functions of such people. By vitiating the Kapha and Medhas, it will produce Pitta and Vata disorders in Jangala places.

The correct treatment will have to take into account the characteristics of location and treating not only the patient but also the land, water and air.

**From the South** – when the wind blows from the South it is correspondingly believed that it has anti-Pitta properties and regulates blood and the Vata. It is good for the eyes and the sensory organs.

While often referring to air pollution on a macro level, there is a tendency to gloss over the kind of pollution that exists on a micro level or on an individual to individual basis. While sitting, talking, dining or interacting with intimacy, using each other's clothes or covers or bed-sheets and personal effects and simple acts of exchange such as garlanding is fraught with the dangers of pollution and infection. The risks inherent in such infection include the possibility of contracting fevers, skin rashes and disease, cough and cold, conjunctivitis, the flu and depending on circumstances even wasting diseases, gastroenteritis, syphilis and gonorrhoea. It may be borne in mind that the mode of spread for the plague was exactly the kind of interaction outlined above.

**Vitiated Air** – Air is as important to humans as the food that they eat and, therefore, to be imbibed in a pure and unpolluted form, if health is to be maintained in a state of equilibrium. Yet, in terms of how easily pollution can occur, air is the most easily polluted, followed by Jala or water, Desha or area and country, and finally Kala. In Ayurveda, it is believed that Adharma, and the malefic influence of the Grahas on humans is a major causative factor in the vitiation of air.

The term 'vitiated air' applies to all abnormal atmospheric conditions – stillness and lack of breeze or stronger than normal winds, abnormally hot or cold or dry or humid winds for that particular region, an excess of *Abhishyandi*, a virulent atmosphere, or one that is loaded with chemicals and toxic fumes, air that is full of noise or is dusty, sandy or smelly.

Vitiated air is a major factor for the insidious onset of disease that may not appear life threatening in the short run, but causes a chronic weakening and so shortens lifespans.

The causative factors for such pollution must be identified and eradicated while proper treatment for its effects is given. Treatment must utilise measures such as fasting, continence, use of digestive stimulants, tonics for the body, treatment for the Doshas and their removal from the body. *Langhana, Langhana Pachana* and *Doshavasechana* are possible lines of treatment. So is *Daiva Vyapasraya* and shifting to more congenial surroundings or salubrious climates. Nutrition and quality of water helps and pure, hot water in itself provides benefits. On a transcendental plane, recitation of Mantras, performing Yogas, the Mangala Pata, Bali. Homa and Havans, are all useful in combating ill effects. Sound pollution, whether caused by factories or traffic, does produce stress and strain and will render the physical being to become prone to disease, and therefore, must be prevented.

# PART C

## NATURE CURE

### *(NISARGOPACHARAM)*

# 39

# INTRODUCING NISARGOPACHARAM

Man is a microcosm of Nature, and so, the Panchmahabhutas, namely, *Prithvi, Ap, Tejo, Vayu* and *Akasha*, that are the very stuff of Nature are also what every human being is made of. Health being a normal condition of for humans, ill-health and disease may thus be considered as aberrations of Nature. Extending this further, all aberrations, whether they are natural or on account of personal habits, or whether they are imposed upon one, are likely to promote diseases. Therefore, inhaling polluted air and drinking polluted water, or consuming improper food and an improper lifestyle of keeping odd hours or promiscuity or poor behaviour by way of disrespect for teachers, elders and God and neglect of Sadvritta and Sadacharas, all enhance the risk of contracting disease.

Nature Cure is treatment of disease by employing natural components, not by medicine and is part and parcel of Ayurveda which has developed a number of methods such as *Lepa* (unguentum), *Vasti* (enema), *Abhyanga* (massage) and *Upavasa* (fasting and control of the diet) for treating ill-health.

Panchakarma therapy employs Nature Cure and the five steps used by those who adhere to the Charaka school of thought are:

1. *Vamana Karma* – Emesis therapy
2. *Virechana Karma* – Purgation therapy
3. *Niruha Vasti* – Decoctions for enemas

4. *Anuvasana Vasti* – Oily enemas with nutritional capability
5. *Nasya* – Errhine therapy

As per Sushrutha's school of thought, the two enema therapies are clubbed together, but blood letting is included as he considered *Rakta* (blood) to be one of the Doshas.

Prior to conducting this line of treatment, some preparatory procedures must be applied, and these are *Snehana Karma* (oleation therapy) and *Swedana Karma* (sudation therapy).

Once the entire treatment is concluded, the patient is put on a special dietary regimen to stoke digestive fires. Thereafter, some medicine may be prescribed.

This therapy is of special benefit to people whose bodies are in a run-down condition because of the stresses of a fast-paced life. Typically, those whose lives have been ruled by hurry, worry, excitement and tension; those who rarely find time to sit at ease for their meals and who have, as a consequence, developed conditions of stomach ulcers, gastric upsets and such disorders. Also for those reporting high blood pressure and diabetes.

In today's context, an important fact to take note of is that Nature Cure does not require large facilities or huge hospital complexes. It also does not require complex and expensive equipment or machines. This means that nature treatments impose very little by way of financial burden on the patient.

# 40

# HYDROTHERAPY

Water constitutes nearly eighty per cent of our bodies and is an absolute necessity for all humans, being as important as air for our survival. This water and fluid content of our bodies is called *Apbhuta* in the terminology of Ayurveda and happens to be one of the five main or Panchmahabhutas.

In addition to the need to drink water regularly to replenish it in our bodies, water is also essential as a cleanser, to wash the body or clothes or our habitats. It is also used for treatments of all kinds.

It is used extensively in Nature Cure, and starting with some of the basic therapies, this chapter will explore some treatments that are part and parcel of Hydrotherapy.

**Hip Baths**

**The Cold Hip Bath** – After exercise, Yogasana and Sooryanamaskara, the patient is made to sit in a tub of water which is three-quarters full. He or she sits so that only the part of his or her body below the waist is submerged in the water. The feet, the upper torso and the legs, for the most part, are kept dry. The water should be at a temperature of between 18 to 24 degrees centigrade and between 4 to 6 gallons of water should be sufficient. The patient is then washed all over his body with a cloth dipped in hot water.

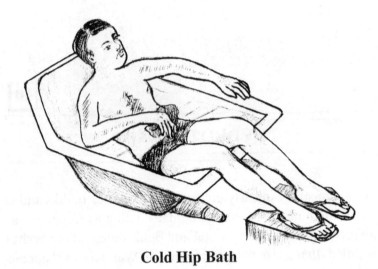

**Cold Hip Bath**

If the patient is in a debilitated condition this treatment can be given in bed, employing a suitable vessel for soaking the hip. The cold hip bath is beneficial for –

1. Cases of obesity, constipation and indigestion
2. Treating piles, ailments connected with the liver and the spleen
3. Pregnancy
4. Prostate enlargement
5. Cases of male impotency and female sterility
6.. All diseases, in a general way

It should not, however, be employed in case of diarrhoea, dysentery, fever, during menses or if the patient is suffering from a backache.

**The Hot Hip Bath** – This requires a specialised tub meant for the purpose. After drinking one or two glasses of water, the patient sits in the tub of water heated to between 40 and 45 degrees centigrade. A cold water pack or cold compress is applied to his head and care should be taken not to massage the abdomen. After this hip bath, the patient should take a shower. The hot hip bath is beneficial for –

1. Cases of delayed menses
2. Relieving burning sensations in the urinary tract
3. Relieving pain caused by haemorrhoids
4. Relieving pain in the anal region
5. Relieving pain in the pelvic region
6. Treating sciatica
7. Providing relief for backaches

The hot hip bath should not, however, be employed in case the patient is suffering from hypertension or weakness due to fever.

**Precaution must be taken** to keep the patient from exposure to cold immediately after the bath and the treatment should be immediately terminated if the patient complains of weakness or giddiness during it.

# MUDBATHS AND PADA PRAKSHALANA

Pada Prakshalana is the term for bathing the feet to bring relief from pain and induce a feeling of freshness to the body. It is done by pouring cold water on the feet, for between five and ten minutes.

**Mud Treatment** – The composition of mud is Panchbhautic, just as is the composition of man. Therefore, its application can restore to an extent, the deficiency in the bhutas of one's body. Applying mud and then taking the additional benefit of sunlight by sun bathing is stimulating.

**The Mudbath** – A mudpack is applied to the patient from head to toe, after which he or she is made to sit out in the sun for between half an hour to an hour. Thereafter, the patient takes a cold water bath or in case feeling chill, a hot water bath. The mud bath is beneficial for –

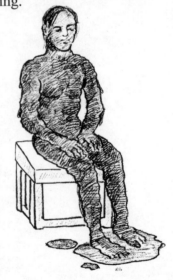

**Mudbath**

1. Increasing blood circulation
2. Enhancing the beauty, colour and lustre of skin
3. Relieving skin ailments such as psoriasis, leprosy, leucoderma and urticaria (*Sita Pitta*)

**The mud** which is used should be of the black soil variety and free from any pollution. Such mud is dried and powdered and preserved in blocks, pending use.

**Mudpacks** – Local applications of mud on the body are called mudpacks. Mudpacks can be made by dipping a thick cloth of size 10"× 6"× 1" in water first and then into mud, which it should absorb. This may then be applied appropriately.

The pack can be applied to the abdomen for between fifteen to thirty minutes. In cold weather, the patient should be kept warm by covering him or her with a rug. This brings about the following benefits–

1. It alleviates indigestion
2. Brings relief to the gut and improves its motility

Mudpacks may also be applied to the head for the benefits of–

1. Relieving headaches
2. Providing cooling relief

**Facial Mudpacks** – This may be applied on the face for thirty minutes, after which it is washed off with water. Its benefits–

1. Removing pimples, blackheads and cleansing the skin
2. Arresting skin discolouration and restoring skin colour
3. Enhancing the beauty of the face itself

**Mudpacks for Eye treatment** – Mudpacks may be used for the eyes for periods of between twenty and thirty minutes to treat–

1. Conjunctivitis (*Abhishyanda*)
2. Redness in the eyes
3. Itching in the eyes
4. Short-sightedness
5. Long-sightedness
6. Glaucoma

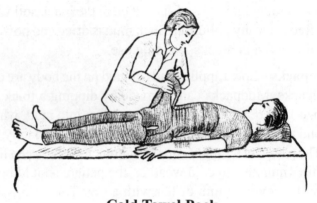

**Cold Towel Pack**
Soothes the nerves and improves circulation in the abdomen

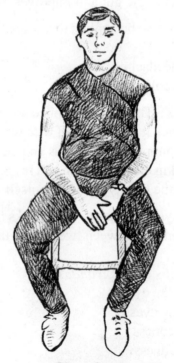

**Chest Pack**
Useful for treating colds, coughs, bronchitis and fever

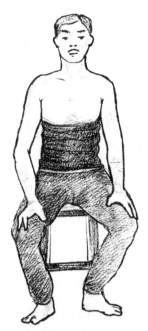

**Abdominal Pack**
Useful for treating gastritis, jaundice and constipation

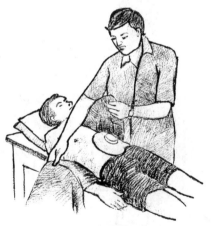

**Towel Pack**
Useful for treating kidney diseases and controlling albumin and urea

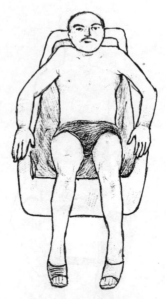

**Cold Spinal Bath**
Useful for multiple conditions

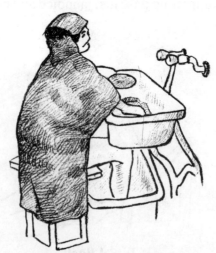

**Foot and Arm Bath**
Useful for treating gout, rheumatism and obesity

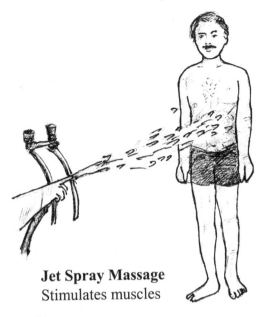

**Jet Spray Massage**
Stimulates muscles

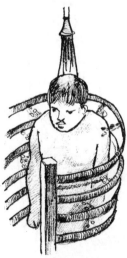

**Circular Jet Spray
Massage**
Stimulates muscles

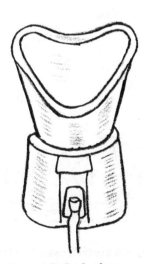

**Steam Inhalation
Equipment**
For use in treating colds,
sinusitis and asthma

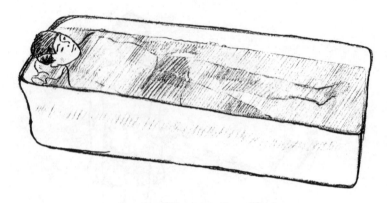

**Neutral Immersion Bath**
Stimulates the skin and kidneys
and is beneficial for arthritis and paralysis

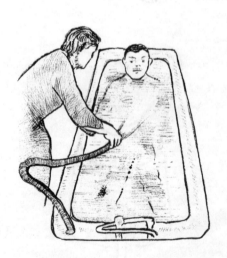

**Underwater Pressure Massage**
Useful as a relaxant of muscles

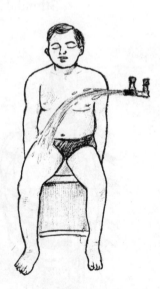

**Affusion Bath**

# 42

# STEAM INHALATION AND SUDATION THERAPY

Steam Inhalation usually involves equipment by way of a facial sauna but can be performed even if the apparatus is not available. Water in a vessel is simply heated to steaming point and kept on a table or stand in front of which the patient sits on a stool. The patient then bends forward with a towel spread over his head and around the vessel to stop the steam from escaping, and inhales the steam for between five and ten minutes, taking care that steam does not affect the eyes. Such inhalation provides–

1. Relief from a Cold
2. Improvement in condition during an attack of Diptheria
3. Relief for Sinusitis
4. Brings up any phlegm stuck in the throat and thorax
5. Relief for headaches
6. Improvement in condition of Asthmatics

**Sudation Therapy** – A steam room has to be constructed for conducting sudation therapy – making the body sweat for flushing out toxins. The patient sits inside this steam room, where the heat of the steam makes him sweat. The duration is usually for ten to fifteen minutes, or per individual preference or simply until sweat appears. The patient should have a cold bath both before and after the procedure, and should then rest for approximately half an hour.

**Precaution must be taken** if the patient complains of weakness or giddiness during the treatment, in which case, the patient should be immediately removed from the room and given some water to drink, followed by a cold bath.

Sudation therapy provides relief and benefits for the following conditions –

1. Arthritis
2. Skin diseases
3. Diseases of the nerves
4. Diseases of the urinary tract
5. Headaches and migraines
6. For a number of other ailments

Sudation therapy is contraindicated and should never be conducted on people with –

1. Heart disease
2. High blood pressure
3. Chronic weakness or debility
4. Fevers

# 43

# SAUNA BATHS

Sauna Baths are given in a wooden room or enclosure designed specially for this purpose, with steam being generated by the action of water on pumice stone kept in the room. Turkish baths employ different systems of generating steam and are designed to hold more people, but the end objective for both Saunas and Turkish baths is the same – providing beneficial heat and steam to the body. It is important for one who wants to use these facilities to be properly hydrated, so it is a good idea to drink some water beforehand. While in the chamber, it is customary to have a massage. The bather, once sufficiently warmed, should then come out for a bath before proceeding for a second round till such time as he or she is streaming with sweat. Then it is time to take a thirty-minute rest with a drink of lemon juice in cold water for re-hydration.

Sauna baths are beneficial in case of –
1. Rheumatoid arthritis
2. Bilious disorders
3. Obesity and for those who want to lose weight
4. Sciatica
5. Backaches and back conditions
6. Chronic indigestion

Such baths should **not** be attempted by those who suffer from–
1. Heart disease
2. Diabetes Mellitus
3. An emaciated condition
4. Hypertension
5. Fever
6. Kidney disease

**Sponge Baths** – These may be given to persons, too weak except to recline. Some equipment is required for a proper sponge bath, and consists of – large absorbent towels known as Turkish towels, a bucket, Turkish blows,Turkish cloth and a rubber sheet for spreading on the bed. Concluded quickly, the sponge bath is actually a rub-down for the bather.

**Cold Friction Baths** – A hot water bag, gloves, aprons, a blanket and a bucket of water is required for giving a cold friction bath. The bather lies down on a table, face upwards. Assistants dip their gloves in water and then run their gloved hands over the bather's body, providing a friction massage from head to toe, before covering the body with the blanket to preserve heat. After a short span, the bather then takes a cold bath.

Cold friction baths provide the following benefits –
1. Relief in case of high blood pressure
2. Bring down fevers
3. Stimulate the nerves
4. Relief from fatigue, fever and pain
5. Promotes good eyesight
6. Soothes and relaxes, and so, acts as a soporific

**Vibro Massage** – This is a massage administered with a machine that vibrates. Talcum powder should be sprinkled on the body before the massage. A vibro massage that lasts

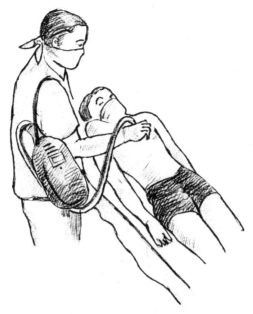

**Vibro Massage**

for half an hour is very soothing, besides stimulating the nervous and circulatory systems.

However, **neither friction baths nor vibro massages** should be undertaken by those who –

1. are pregnant
2. are menstruating
3. have skin disease
4. are fasting
5. have diarrhoea
6. have dysentery
7. have just undergone Panchakarma therapy

# 44

# MASSAGE

Massage is a very important part of the process of treatment in Ayurveda. Massage pacifies the Vata, a propelling force. Oil is invariably applied during massage; often massage is combined with an oil bath. The benefits of an oil bath are as enumerated –

1. It relieves pain
2. It relieves fatigue, soothes and rejuvenates
3. Regular massage delays the onset of old age
4. It promotes good eyesight
5. It keeps the body supple and lends it strength and sturdiness
6. It is a promoter of good sleep

Oil, when applied to the head, ears and feet, has a synergistic effect with the massage.

**Udvartana** – This is a massaging technique that employs a dry powder called *Sudarshana Choorna,* to treat obesity and problems with phlegm. Udvartana begins from the feet and works upwards. This way of massaging, when performed in the reverse order, is called *Pratilomagati.* Prakriti Chikitsa or Nature Cure employs Ayurvedic styles of massage.

**Abhyanga** – Massaging techniques that employ oils are called Abhyanga (oil massage). The person who is to be massaged, after removal of clothes, lies down on a Abhyanga table, or

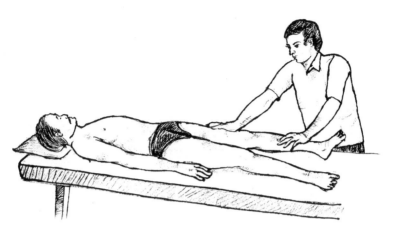

**Oil Massage**

*Droni,* as it is called. The Droni is made from a single log of teak. In the case of Vata and Kapha disorders, the oil to be applied is warmed, whereas in the case of disorders of the Pitta, oil at normal temperature is applied. The massage takes place in the *Anulomagati* way, that is, starting from the head and working downwards. The massage is done with a soft touch, as applying heavy pressures while massaging will produce Vata. There can be any of seven postures employed for the massage, which lasts fifteen to twenty minutes, during which warm oil is applied in the ears. On conclusion, the person rests for fifteen minutes before taking a bath.

The Abhyanga massage is not recommended for treating obesity and problems with phlegm. Nor is it suitable during bouts of indigestion or after Panchakarma therapy. Its benefits are similar to the ones listed earlier, in the case of the oil bath.

# 45

# FASTING

Fasting should be the prelude to all treatments conducted in the manner of Ayurveda and Nature Cure. Fasting purifies and detoxifies the seven Dhatus present in the body, and even children, pregnant women and the aged should fast before such treatment.

Food serves three purposes, namely –
1. Shodhana – eliminative or as roughage
2. Santarpana – energy producing
3. Growth enhancing

In equilibrium, the three together promote growth and a feeling of well being. But, either due to the presence of morbid material, or due to the vitiation of the Doshas, when unbalance occurs, it causes illness and discomfort. Fasting helps with the process of natural balancing.

The duration one must fast is determined by one's physician's advice, or at least until some symptoms enumerated below have been eradicated. These are –
1. Feelings of lack of taste
2. Smell in the mouth
3. Coating on the tongue
4. Abdominal cramps
5. Giddiness
6. Nausea and vomiting
7. Fatigue

During the fast, it is important not to tax oneself either physically or mentally. Fasting need not always be total. It can often be a light fast, when small quantities of beneficial foods can be eaten. Such foods would consist of juices, fruits, butter-milk and vegetables such as carrots, some varieties of beans, bitter gourd and cabbage, or their extracts. These must be chewed thoroughly before swallowing. At least a quarter of one's stomach capacity must be allowed to remain empty. This constitutes a Satvic diet, to which earlier references have been made. The consent of the physician may be sought for items such as coconut water, barley, pineapple, bananas, almonds, lemon, horse gram and karela.

Ghee and butter, chapatis, rice, dal, curd, meat and beverages like tea and coffee are preferably not to be taken, or if at all, to be kept to the barest minimum. Alcohol, deep fried foods, condiments such as mustard and pepper, cocoa are taboo.

One must take precaution against the build up of excess uric acid in the blood, uric acid being the contributing factor for conditions such as gout. It should be borne in mind that a variety of common food items contain oxalates that give rise to stones and produce excesses of uric acid. These are – tomatoes, the chiku fruit, cashew-nut, cucumber, black grapes which are rich in oxalates, and pumpkin, mushroom and brinjal which are rich in uric acid.

Water in plenty is good and one may drink between one and three glasses in a Padmasana posture, well before treatment begins. Other preparations should include breathing deeply while in an erect posture, thorough evacuation of faeces and urine, bathing and some rest.

After meals and evacuation, one should adopt the Vajrasana posture for a few minutes and should sleep in a simple bed. Sleep after meals is recommended, so is lying down on one's abdomen. One should cleanse the mind of all evil thoughts.

# 46

# EXERCISE
# (VYAYAMA)

Vyayama is the old Sanskrit word for exercise, and in Nature Cure, exercising is considered to be an essential part of the recovery process. Exercise is natural to all animals, and human beings are no exception. Exercise not only tones the muscles, but also our internal systems, whether the cardiovascular and the circulatory system or the digestive system.

Vyayama can take many forms, from the light to the hectic. Walking, running, performing the Asanas and Yogasana, swimming, weight-lifting, and training, and participating in sports. During recovery from an illness however, the strenous should naturally be avoided until fitness builds up.

Walking is an excellent way to start with, gradually building up to cover distances of more than a mile. Most people should target themselves to be able to cover three miles in due course. Ideally, the route one takes should be through pleasant, natural surroundings and offer stimulation for the senses.

Exercise should be regular and become a part of our daily or weekly regimen, coupled with meals at regular times and a healthy and nourishing diet that avoids toxic foods. Exercise arrests the aging process.

We should eat to live and not live to eat. All food intake should be based upon one's own level of exercising. For athletes and others on strenous routines, supplemental foods should be taken. For all, however, fasting once a week is beneficial, and artificial diets and dieting fads to be avoided.

# 47

# ENEMA THERAPY
# (VASTI KARMA)

Vasti Karma, which is a therapy based on the administration of enemas, is believed to be a very effective way of treating disorders of the Vata. The large intestine is the seat of Vata and enemas act there directly. Ayurveda and Nature Cure use slightly different approaches to washing the area.

Equipment, by way of an enema can, nozzles and piping, is required for administrating an enema.

In Ayurveda, the patient is made to lie in the left lateral position with his or her left leg extended and the right one flexed. The enema nozzle is then smeared with oil or any oily substance and passed through the rectum. Then, between two and four pints of plain, hot water is passed into the gut, for retaining for five to ten minutes. The patient can then take a short stroll before evacuating the contents of his guts, faeces and water in the lavatory.

While the process used in Nature Cure is similar, the difference is that in this case the patient is made to lie down in the right lateral position and the hot water used contains salt.

The benefits of such enemas are clearing the bowels and relieving a constipated condition. In case the patient has reported with dysentery, then water at a temperature of 18 degrees centigrade should be used. Patients with piles should be given water at between 40 and 42 degrees centigrade. For those who suffer from amoebiasis, a neem decoction should be mixed with the enema water as this will kill most of the organisms responsible.

# 48

# VAGINAL DOUCHE
# (YONI PRAKSHALANA)

Prakshalana is the term for the process of applying douches. Douches are similar to enemas in the way that they are applied, except that they are applied to the vaginal canal and not to the lower part of the alimentary tract. Hot, warm, lukewarm and cold water are all used depending upon the case being treated, but the water is invariably applied at a pressure.

The patient lies down on her back, with a bed pan under the thighs and posterior, which are slightly raised. Water at slight pressure is applied through a nozzle in the vaginal canal, care being taken to place this nozzle behind the uterus.

The douche, besides cleansing the vagina, stimulates its mucus membrane and improves circulation in the pelvic region.

**Cold Douche** – When there is menorrhagia or excess bleeding in the vagina, the cold douche is applied for between ten and fifteen minutes. As the term implies, a cold douche employs cold water. This tones up the uterus and arrests bleeding. It also pacifies any burning sensations there may be in the canal and relieves any itching or swelling in the urinary tract.

**Hot Douche** – the term for this in Nature Cure is *Ushna Prakshalana*. The water should be at 40 degrees centigrade. This is effective as a pain reliever, for cases of salpingitis, oophoritis and endometritis.

Douches must not be administered if the patient is pregnant, although they are sometimes used just before delivery to dilate the cervix. Often, both hot and cold irrigation is employed to stimulate the pelvic organ.

# 49

# THE SUN BATH

Sunlight is vital for both animal and plant life, and so, sunbathing is a part of the Nature Cure process.

**Radiation from the Sun** – In addition to the visible spectrum (VIBGYOR) that radiates from the sun, its radiation consists of the infra-red and the ultraviolet. While excesses could be harmful, the **infra-red** provides heat and is good for people in a chilled condition. It is a natural pain reliever. It relieves swelling of the tissues and soothes and relaxes them. The **ultraviolet** range helps the body synthesise vitamins in the skin, notably Vitamin D, and assists in the formation and maintenance of our bones, and acts to prevent diseases such as rickets.

Sunbathing, therefore, has been an activity practised by early civilisations across the globe and many references can also be found in Roman texts, for example. In addition to the vital benefits mentioned above, sunbathing also provides the following–

1. Growth and maintenance of teeth
2. Assists growth of hair
3. Improves respiration
4. Its soothing action is good for lowering high blood pressure
5. Assists kidney function

6. Heals wounds on the skin
7. Makes blood less acidic, provides alkalis to the blood
8. Nourishes pregnant women

A number of diseases are prevalent when there is a lack of sunlight. These include tuberculosis, rickets, pneumonia, physical deformity and a high incidence of death among children, and the flourishing of epidemics.

It is best to be bare-bodied while taking a sun bath.

**Precaution must be taken,** however, against exposure to too much sunlight in locations where the sunlight is very strong. Excessive ultraviolet radiation can burn skin and be harmful. The first harmful effect is to the eyes, where prolonged exposure leads to the formation of cataracts. It is advisable, therefore, to keep the head covered and the eyes shut or covered with dark glasses while sunbathing. Excessive sunlight can also cause skin cancers, especially among fair-skinned people. Thus, it is advisable to sunbathe in the mornings and evenings when the sunshine is less harsh. It is also advisable to stop sunbathing when one feels burning sensations on the skin, or fatigued and sleepy. A cold water bath is the best way of relief from sunburn.

# PART D

---

# THE SCIENCE OF YOGA

## *(YOGA VIJNANAM)*

---

# 50

# HOW AYURVEDA RELATES TO YOGA
# (SWASTHAVRITTA VIJNANAM)

Yoga is a science that is quite similar to, although independant of, Ayurveda, in terms of the basic principles.

Like Ayurveda -

- Yoga believes in recognising the person as a combination of mind, body, soul and senses.
- Yoga advises methods and practices which are natural and in harmony with our system.
- The ultimate goal of both Ayurveda and Yoga is to achieve Moksha (Salvation) by living a balanced life.
- Although the ultimate goal or meaning of Yoga is to connect the soul with God, it draws upon processes and principles developed by Ayurveda, such as Satvic diets and lifestyles prescribed by the latter.
- Yoga prescribes following a regimen and has formulated near-identical rules and regulations to Ayurveda, governing non-violence, social conduct, ethics, and beneficial practices for maintenance of health and curing disease.
- Yoga is a process or discipline that aims to stop or remove animal desires from the mind. The process involves rules to be followed in eating, living, physical exercise, breathing exercises, controlling the senses,

concentrating and strengthening the mind. Ayurveda corroborates these practices as the best for preventing disease and maintaining good health.

## Yoga

The practices or process of Yoga are very beneficial for maintenance of health. Yoga is holistic in nature and so takes into account the state of the mind for which it has developed procedures. Thus, Yoga helps to maintain both physical and mental health, which cannot be done by either taking pills or drinking potions. But complex states such as one's mind can be controlled by the correct practice of Yoga, whose ultimate purpose is to strengthen the mind. Yoga helps one overcome mental depression as well as attain equilibrium between body and soul. Yoga increases the capacity to work and benefits the brain by increasing retention power and memory.

Yoga can take various forms and this subject is dealt with in more detail in Chapter 53 that follows. Basically, it employs two main formats, *Rajayoga,* which is behaviourial, and *Hathayoga,* which is physical. These, in turn, employ various *Yogasanas* (physical postures), *Satkarmas* (six therapies for purifying the body and increasing vitality of life, thereby decreasing risk of disease) and *Pranayama* (breathing exercises).

The Asanas and Pranayamas increase the blood and air circulation and rejuvenate the body. For example, while performing Sarvangasana, blood circulation in the thyroid gland increases, which in turn strengthens the thyroid gland. Similarly, Shirsasana increases blood circulation to the head, neck, and brain.

Likewise, there are others that produce massage-like effects on the stomach, intestines, liver, pancreas, gall bladder and kidneys. Different postures attained during Yogasanas exert pressure on these organs in individual ways, at particular sites, resulting in regulated blood circulation to these. Yoga is known to cause reflex actions and feedback reactions, which affects and improves the functioning of organs. Yoga is not a mystery, as some tend to think, and its effect has been evaluated by various physiological and pharmacological studies.

The vision of Yoga is encapsulated in the ancient scriptures, and so, this text will attempt an examination of numerous such quotes in this and the chapters that follow.

*Yathahi KritsnamVikarajatam Satvrajathmamsi Navyathirchyate|*
*Evameva Kritsanam Vikarajatam|*
*Viswarupena Vathitamatirichya Vaata Pitta Sleshmano Vartante|*
*Samatvam Yoga Uchyate||*

The Geeta says that equanimity must be maintained through joy or misery. This is the philosophy of Nishkama Karma. Yoga maintains equilibrium among one's Satva, Rajas and Tamas.

Both Yoga and Ayurveda are based on striving to balance the factors within one.

**Ayu**

Ayu is the term for lifespan and can take four forms, differing from person to person:

1. *Sukhayu* - That part of life that is spent with pleasantness and in good health
2. *Dukhayu* - the part that is miserable
3. *Hitayu* - the part that is devoted to society and good causes
4. *Ahitayu* - the part spent on oneself

Both Yoga and Ayurveda recommend that at least a part of life should be spent in the Hitayu phase, contributing to the welfare of others.

The terminology used by both to describe human states and situations is the same.

While Ayurveda mainly focuses on the state of health of a person while alive and in the course of life, Yoga focuses on the attainment of salvation and strives to create the impeccable physical and mental states that are required for such fusion with the Ultimate.

# 51

# DESCRIPTIONS OF YOGA
# IN AYURVEDA

Freedom from all types of pain is to attain salvation. Both
Yoga and Ayurveda postulate this. While Ayurveda cautions
one to stay away from suffering, Yoga teaches one to overcome
it. This may be gleaned from the scriptures, some of which
are reproduced here.

*Yoge Mokshe Cha Sarvesham Vedananmavartanam|*
*Moksho Nivritti Vischeshya Yogo Moksha Pravartaka:||*
                              *... {Charaka Shareera, 1:137}*
Yoga can bring about personality changes (*Chitta Vritti
Nirodha*). The mind (*Manas*) and speech is brought under
control. Then, with focus (*Dhyaana*) one can rid one's mind
of negative qualities such as *ahamkara*, *kama*, *krodha* and
*parigraha*. This achievement is the beginning of fusion with
the Brahma and so salvation (*Mukti*).

*Samassenatu    Kaunteyanishta    Jnanasyayapara    -*
*Brahmabhitta|*
*Prashanta Tama Nashochating Kankshati||*
                              *... {Bhagavad Geeta}*
Just as in Ayurveda, Moksha is the final goal of the four
*Purusharthas* (the reason for existing as an adult), so also in
Yoga, which assists in attaining *Parinama* and salvation.

*Satyavadinam Krodha Nivrittam Madya Maithunath|*
*Ahimsa Kamanasyam Prashantam Priyavadinam|*
*Jap - Souch - Param Dhairyam Danam Nityam Tapasminam|*
*Devagobrahmanacharyaguru Buddharchane Ratam||*
*Anrushamshya Pararan Nityam Karunya Vedenam|*
*Samajagarana SwapnamNityam Ksheera Ghratasinam||*
*Deshakala Pramanajnam Yuktijna Maham Krutam|*
*Sastra Charamsankeerna Madyatma Pravanendriyam||*
*Upasitaram Buddhinamsthikanam Jitatumanam||*
*... {Charaka}*

One must adopt the practices (detailed hereunder) to get benefits similar to Acharya Rasayana.

1. Always tell and practise the truth.

2. Never succumb to rage and such negative feelings.

3. Stay away from alcohol.

4. Stay away from illicit sex.

5. Avoid excessive fatigue.

6. Become peace loving, discard aggressive postures.

7. Practise *Japa* (litany) and *Tapas* (penance).

8. Respect teachers, elders and people of learning, irrespective of caste and creed. Respect knowledge and those who posses it.

9. Perform charitable acts.

10. Exhibit kindness.

11. Stick to proper schedules, sleep in time.

12. Wake up at Brahminhurta, the time when the faculties are at their sharpest

13. Meditate regularly.

14. Practise what is taught in the litanies you recite.

*Atmendriya Manoarthanam Sannikarshat Pravartate|*
*Sukha Dukha Manarambhadatmasthe Manasisthire||*
*Nivartate Ladu BhayamVasitwam Chopa Jayate|*
*Sa Shareerasya YogaJnastvam Yoga Mrushayo Viduhu||*

Happiness and sorrow are functions of our *Indriyas* (personality), through which we derive knowledge about the soul (*Atmajnana*) through our Manas (mental faculties or powers of reasoning). If the mind is connected to the soul, then feelings such as misery will not occur.

Yogis call this detailed analysis from Ayurveda, *Nivritti*.

Both schools give the mind its due importance for affecting well-being. While Chitta Vritti Nirodha and control of the mind is aimed at in Yoga through adherence to Yama, Niyama and Rasayana, Ayurveda deals with corrections to the Vata as the active force behind the functioning of the brain, the nervous system and connected cells.

Both schools are one on the subject of what is proscribed or unacceptable behaviour, or, as they term it, *Adharma*.

# 52

# THE ROLE OF YOGA AS A
# SAFEGUARD FOR HEALTH

Yoga and Ayurveda are one in the belief that the health of the individual is all-important. To draw upon a Sloka that is common to both practices-

*Dhoutirvastistatheneti Navliki Tratakam Tathaa|*
*Kapaala Bhati Schaitani Shat karmani Samaacharet||*

*{Ghoranda 1 / 12}*

This advocates the purification of the body by performing the *S(h)at Karmas.* As adopted in Ayurveda, the Sat Karmas reduce the state of disease in the body and pacify the Rajas and Tamas. As adopted in Yoga, the Sat Karmas purify the Sharira (body) and the Manas (mind).

Both practices are aimed at achieving a state of *Prasannata* in the individual. Equivalents for Prasannata in English are happiness, contentment, joy and beatification. A state of Prasannata is a state of health and Ayurveda looks to balancing the Doshas, Dhatus, Mala, Agni and Indriyas to achieve this. Yoga teaches that the adoption of *Yama* and *Niyama* (codes and regimes) result in *Saralta* (calm) and *Vimalta* (control) in the individual. These very similar concepts are basic to achieving joy and, thus, a state of health.

Muscles, tendons, ligaments and the Prishtha (the back and the spinal column) are all part of body tissue and the better their tone and the stronger they are, the more one feels well. Yoga exercises these systematically and carefully, thus toning them up and improving health. This harmonises with the importance of exercise in Ayurveda. The practise of Yoga also allows the Tristhambas of food, sleep and sexual continence to achieve their correct balance, besides toning up the body's own disease resistance systems. *Prajnaparadha* is the opposite of Prasannata and both sciences hold the condition responsible for ill health. Practicing Yoga removes Prajnaparadha.

**Benefits of Yoga**
The benefits of Yoga have been enumerated in a Sloka from the Hatha Yoga Pradeepika -
*Swaa Akaasa Pleeha Kushtam, Kapharoga Scha Vimshati|*
*Dhouti Karma Prabhavena Prayathny Vana Shamshaya:||*
*Kaooaala Sodhini Chaiva Diva Drushti Pradayini|*
*Urdhajatrughatan Rogan Netirashu Nihanticha||*
*Gulma Pleehadaram Chaapi Vato Pitta Kaphodbhava:||*
*Vasti Karma Prabhaa Vena Kheeyante Sakalaamaya:*
*Mandagni Sandeepana Paachanaadi Sandaapika|*
*Nandakarisadaiva|*
*Aptopadesha Madeshonicha Hatakriyaa Mauleya Cha Nanli:||*

The explanation for the Sloka needs to be elaborated in the modern context. The 1936 Nobel Prize winner, Seely, was the first person in our modern day to enunciate the growing realisation that perturbed thinking, brought about by fear, sorrow, stress and constant adrenaline secretions due to over-stimulation brings about a diseased condition. When someone is excited, it results in an increase in adrenaline which causes the blood pressure to soar. A cycle will then occur. First, the stage of alarm or panic reactions, then the stage of resistance, and finally a state of exhaustion. This lowers the basal metabolic rate or B.M.R., as it is commonly known. Continual such cycles or a bad diet then causes a thickening of the arterial wall (Arteriosclerosis), which leads to chronic hypertension and the cycle repeating itself. This is a main cause of heart diseases such as angina pectoris, congestive cardiac failure and cardiac asthma.

On the other hand, it is now proven through any number of tests on the ECG that meditation increases the basal metabolic rate and reduces the strain on the heart.

When fear, sorrow, stress and anxiety intrude upon our thinking and produce mental restlessness, or in the terminology of Yoga, mental Kshoba and restlessness of the Brahma, this shows up on EEC readings. Meditation pacifies the brain, as is evident in the generation of alpha waves on the EEC monitors. Yoga, with its emphasis on meditation, is thus a health promoter for the body, as well as the mind.

With Yoga, both mental efficiency and activity improve. Tests for memory, mental performance and mental fatigue, all exhibit remarkable improvement. Tests also show that Yoga significantly improves the body's internal temperature control mechanism and has a positive impact on blood chemistry, serum lipids and plasma catecholamines, decreasing the harmful ones. It retards degeneration of tissues and the aging process, and stimulates the production of antibodies and recovery.

In the modern world, with pollution in air and water and declining nutrition in foods due to adulteration and synthetic production, health threats abound. Yoga and meditation are proven to have beneficial effects on health and this is gaining worldwide recognition and popularity.

*Matirvacha: Karma Sukhanubandham, Satya Vidheya Vishada Cha Buddhi|*

*... {Charaka}*

Yoga preserves and protects health by producing antibodies in the blood and by regulating the body and mind, explains Charaka.

*Jnanam Tapastatparata Cha Yoge Yashyastatam Nannu*
*Patantirogaa:|*
*Nitymhita Ahara Viharasevee Sameekshakari*
*Vishayevaskta:||*

                                 *... {Charaka}*

Achieve your desires through the practice of Yoga. Yama and Niyama are the most important two out of the eight Angas or subdivisions of Yoga. They deal with the mental aspects of Yoga and observing these leads to a clarity of mind and purpose, a purity, if you will, that is essential before attaining Samadhi. Another equivalent of Yama in Sanskrit is *Ahimsa*, or benevolence to all. *Niyam* a means to follow principles or to follow a discipline.

## The Paribhasha of Yama

*Dehendriyeshu Vairagyam Yama Etyuchyate Budha:|*
*Trishikhi Bhranopashad||*
Practising Yama leads to Vairagya of the body and Indriyas.

*Abyasenatu Kaunteya Vairagyena Cha Grihyate|*
Practising Yama leads to removal of Prajnaparadha

The root cause of all disease is Prajnaparadha, which produces Vibrahmsa of Dhee, Dhriti and Raga. Vairagya dispels these.

*Dyyato Vihayan Pumatisangastheshupa Jayate|*

# 53

# THE ORIGIN AND STRUCTURE OF YOGA

Yoga, as a Word or *Shabda*, occurs frequently in the ancient texts, the Shastras, Upanishads and the Sutras. It is often used in a variety of contexts and with different meanings whose Sanskrit equivalent could be any of Sambadha, Sannahara, Upaya, Sangati, Jnana and Yukti.

Patanjali, the founder of Yoga, described it as *"Yoga Chittavritti Nirodha:"*, literally that the mind has its say for all the activities of man. Yoga makes the mind focus on its Soul.

Later Katopanishad had this to say about Yoga, *"Taam Yogamiti Manyante Sthira Mindriya Dharanaam"*, meaning that Yoga turns the mind from worldly distractions towards the inner world of one's soul, bringing mind, senses and strength under control.

Thus, Yoga developed as a technique through which man exercised control over his physical and mental being, to attain hitherto unachieved states of bliss and to be able to conjecture on God or The Supreme Soul, the *Parmatma*, and to dwell upon the creation and existence of this world.

### Astanga (Eight-faceted) Yoga
Yoga is known as Astanga or eight-faceted Yoga and these eight facets are enumerated as under:

1. Yama
2. Niyama
3. Asana
4. Pranayama
5. Pratyahara
6. Dharana
7. Dhyana
8. Samadhi

**Yama** - As referred to earlier, Yama stands for Ahimsa, benevolence to all living beings, respect and tolerance and objectivity in all feeling, doing and observing. Gautam Buddha said "*Ahimsa Paramo Dharma*", meaning Ahimsa is the supreme religion. Patanjali said, "*Ahimsa Pratishtayam Tatsnmidhou Vairatyaga:|*" that is, when animals bade farewell to Ahimsa, they chose the route to enmity. Practise of Yama requires -

**Satya (Truth):**
> *Ahimsa Pratishtayam Kriya Phalasrayatam |*
> *... {Patanjali}*

One must always speak and think truthfully. Such speech is completely with Dharma and others should not be offended.

**Asteya (Abstaining from Stealing):**
> *Ahimsa Pratishtayam Sarvaratnopa Sthanam |*
> *... {Patanjali}*

One will never be happy stealing from others or being jealous of others goodness, riches and lifestyles. One who overcomes such acts is showered with precious stones.

**Brahmacharya (Celibacy):**

*Smaranam Kirtanam Kalehi: Prekshanam Guhya Bhashanam|*
*Sankalpodhya Vasayascha Kriya Nispathi Revacha|*
*Ethan Maithuna Mastangam Pravadanti Manishana:||*

Brahmacharya or true celibacy is when the mind fuses with the Parabrahma or the highest levels of consciousness. Retaining semen (Veerya) is not Brahmacharya. Brahmacharya would include doing away with:

1. Smarana (thinking about sexual partners)
2. Kirtana (singing about attractions, about ladies)
3. Kelihi (meeting)
4. Prekshana (interacting with other potential partners, other ladies)
5. Guhya Bhashana (coitus and voyeurism)
6. Sankalpa (viewing entertainment with titillating content, e.g. cinema)
7. Adhyavasaya (reading books or discussing or viewing material with pornographic content)
8. Kriya Nispathi

*Brahmacharya Pratishtaya Veeryalabha*, that is, Brahmacharya benefits the semen and life-force.

*Tasmat Shastra Pramante Karya Karya Vyavasthita Jnatva Shastra Vidhanoktam Karma Kar Mihaharsi*, or, having studied the Shastra, one must follow them precisely to get benefits; to do otherwise is the behaviour of animals.

*Edi Varatyaa Samyujyante Pranameva Praskandante|*
*Tavyadratau Ratya Samyujyante Brahmacharyameva||*

Coitus, during daytime is proscribed as it results in depletion of the Ojas, the life-force.

**Rutu Kala:** The purpose of marriage is to sanctify the taking of a partner for the purpose of propagating the race and begetting an heir. Dharma, Artha and Kama are only the intermediate stages to salvation. Therefore, one must not have sex with any other than one's lawfully wedded wife and that too only during Rutu Kala, the period which starts on the fourth day after menstruation and ends on the sixteenth. To derive the benefits of Brahmacharya, one does not need to give up sex altogether. Simply that it is limited to one's wife.

**Aparigraha:** Although enjoyable, many things we do and are addicted to, such as some of the foods that we eat, are not good for us and must be given up. Such items are called *Bhoga.*

*Aparigraha Sthairyajanma Kathamcha Sambodhai|*

A person who is an Aparigraha will understand the past and future happenings in his life.

**Niyama:** Niyama encompasses the five concepts of *Soucha* (cleanliness), *Santosha* (contentment), *Tapas* (penance), *Swadhyaya* and *Iswari Pranidhana.*

Mental or internal cleanliness is known as *Antah Soucha* while bodily cleanliness is known as *Bahi Soucha.* Bahi Soucha was achieved in the traditional way before a session of Yoga by applying mud on the body. This absorbed the dirt on the body and was scrubbed and washed clean. Antah Soucha consisted of disciplining the mind to treat every human being with equality, by focusing on the fact that each one is a product of the Parmatma.

*Santoshadanuttama Sukha Labha|*

To be truly happy and contented is a state of mind that is quite different, for example, from the temporary happiness derived from seeing a cinema or merely being wealthy.

*Vidhinoktera Margena Kricchra Chandra Yanadibhi:|*
*Sareera Soshanam Prahu Stapa Sasta Pa Uttanam||*

One should follow the path of Vrota like *Kriccha and Chandrayana* to be able to control the senses and attain Moksha. This advocates leading an austere life. A sort of *Vrata* or vow.

*Karyendrisiddhirasuddhi Kshaya Staasa:|*

Penance purifies the body, the Indriyas and Antahakarana.

*Swadhyaya Dista Devata Sampryoga:||*

Practise the Vedas and mantras of which the Gayatri Mantra is the root, strictly in accordance to the procedure prescribed in the shastras (Swadyaya). The mantras and the words must be spelt and pronounced properly.

Mantras are recitations and litany which may be either Vaidika (derived from the Veda texts) or Tantrik (derived from the occult). Vaidika mantras may be either Prageeta or Aprageeta while Tantrik mantras may be either Streelinga, Pullinga or Napunsaka Linga (female, male or neuter in gender). Gurus and elders are supposed to provide guidance for their recitation during forms of Yoga such as Rajayoga and the philosophy involved is explained in Mantra Rahasya.

*Kamatos Kamatospi Yatkaromisubhasubhi|*
*Tatsarvam Twayivinyasya Twatparata Yuktaha Karomyoham||*

Akin to the phrase 'labour of love', one should devote one's soul to God and dedicate one's work to Him regardless of whether one's work brings any material gains. Such a person is called Iswari Pranidhana.

*Samadhi Siddhirswareeswara Pranidhanath|*

By practising Yama and Niyama and the Asanas of Yoga, one is able to gain control of one's body, mind and soul, and thereby gain control over disease.

*Hatasya Prathamangtwa Dasanam Poorvamuchate| Tasmatta*
*Dasanam Kuryadarogyam Changa Laghavan||*

One's mental make-up, determination and volition fluctuate from time to time and weaken. This can be controlled by regulating breathing – the inflow and outflow of air to and from the lungs.

When the focus of the practice is on the Antaratma, the inner spirit or soul, it is called *Hathayoga,* and when this focus is on the Atma or one's own mentality, it is called *Rajayoga.*

*Bhrantya Bahumata Dhwante Rajayogam Janatam|*
*Hat Pradeepikam Dhatte Swatya Ram: Krupakara||*

*Asanam Pran Samrodha: Pratyahara Scha Dharanam*
*Dhyanam Samadhiretani Shadangani Prakirtita||*
*... Upanishad*

To sum up, the Yoga Asanas help to condition the body, the mind and the soul so that one can become impervious to disease, but before Asanas may be practised, a suitable state of mental readiness must be achieved.

# 54

# REGULATIONS FOR YOGA LEARNERS

The Practise of Yoga involves the imposition of considerable self-discipline in one's diet and in the activities one pursues. Yoga is holistic in nature and to develop a grasp of Yoga and to perform the Yoga Asanas (the postures of Yoga) requires a proper physical and mental state at the starting itself.

**Diet:** A Satvic diet is advocated for those who wish to take up Yoga as a practice. Satvic foods have already been discussed in the earlier chapters and will serve as a useful reference in this context. Vegetables should be eaten in moderation, if only on account of the flatulence it is likely to create. To quote from the Slokas -

*Sakena Vardhate Vyadhi:*

Eating large amounts of vegetable increases the risk of disease.

The practitioner's diet must consist of foods that are healthy and provide strength and well-being, foods of the quality comparable to those that are offered to the Gods. Foods that are beneficial include Patola, curd, wheat, milk, sugar and ginger (Shunti). Items that are spicy, pungent, sour or quite salty are to be shunned. Eating foods that are pure assists the mind to become pure.

*Aharasuddhan Satvashuddhi:|*
*Satva Shuddhan Dhruva Smriti:*

*...Upanishad*

This piece of text from the Upanishad says that the foods that generate Rajas and Tamas are taboo. Meat and fat should be eaten in moderation. One must adopt the 'Madhyama Marga' or the middle path in one's behaviour, avoiding, for instance, being overly talkative.

**Vihara:** This is the term for exercise and activity that is as essential for the body as food. Proper exercise and activity also stimulate the mind and the senses with resulting benefits to overall health and physical condition. Generally, though, the levels should be such as to not strain one's capabilities. Undue strain is bad for health. Yoga may be practised at various levels, and so, it is a beneficial activity.

The place for practising Yogasanas must be clean and airy but not windy. Traditionally, such places received a special cleaning with an application of cow-dung, but smooth, flat, cemented surfaces are fine. It is important that Yoga be performed in places, if not fragrant, definitely without any hint of offensive smell or unclean in any way. Never on a roof or in a basement.

Before the conclusion of a session, the practitioner should have worked up a light sweat. At this stage, he or she should rub down the perspiration on the body itself before bathing.

*Jalenasramajatena Gatra Mardanam Charet|*
*Drudhata Laghuta Chaivatenagatrasya Jayate||*

At the conclusion of a session of Yogasanas, the body should not be exposed to breeze for at least an hour, otherwise it will sap strength. Perspiration should be rubbed down on the body itself, before a bath in tepid or hot water. One should not be on a fast or without nourishment when practising Yoga. Ghee, milk and such foods are suitable, and if ghee is taken, it should be at the start of the meal, with the first bowl of food. Yoga practitioners should respect and obey God, their elders, the Gurus and parents.

*Utsahatsaha Sadhairayat Tatta Jnanacha Nischayat|*
*Janasanga Pari Tyagat Shadbhiryoga Prasidhyati||*

While performing Yoga, one's entire focus should be on the
teacher, cutting out all external distractions. One should not
be disheartened with oneself.

*Yuvavruddhoti Vruddhova Vyadhito Duralospiva|*
*Abhyasat Siddhima Pnoti Sarvayogeshwa Tandrita:||*

The practice of Yoga is beneficial for all ages and genders,
from the time when a child is about eight years old. Practise
of the Asanas is not advised for pregnant women, especially
after four months of pregnancy. Although, some specific
techniques, namely Samavritti, Vishamavritti, Ujjayani and
Pranayama should be performed. Kumbhaka is definitely out.
For the elderly who may find other Asanas beyond their
capability, Shirsasana and Surya Namaskara are suitable and
rejuvenating. If possible, they should attempt Uttanupadasana,
Sarvangasana, Halasana, Padmasana, Rechaka, Kumbhaka
and Pranayama. One can practise all the Asanas through
middle age with the benefits of arresting the aging process
and keeping one's faculties sharp. For the ill and the very
weak, some of the asanas and certainly the Pranayama should
be practised. Advice should be sought from an experienced
Yoga teacher.

Regular practise of Yogasana rejuvenates the body. It gives
relief to ailments of both the body and the mind. The propitious
time for these exercises is the Brahmamahurta and they should
never be done in conditions of extreme heat or cold, under
stress, or coupled with sexual urges.

# 55

# THE SUN SALUTATION
# (SURYA NAMASKARA)

The Sun has been conceptualised as a God because of its essential nature for mankind. Accordingly, a proper starting point for the practise of Yoga is the Surya Namaskara or a salutation to the sun.

Yoga posture practises are performed in a series of steps or stages called Vinyasas. Along with the Surya Namaskara, some of them can be performed in two styles – of either nine or seventeen Vinyasas. The others are Vinyasa Krama, Dhyana Krama, Rechaka Krama, Puraka Krama and Trataka Krama.

*Naya Matmabalahinen Labhya:||*

The Sun Salutation provides happiness to the body, the mind and the senses. Happiness is essential for achieving health, longevity, and ultimately, Moksha.

*"Bhadram Karne Bhisrunuyamadeva:|*
*Bhadram Pashye Makshibhirya-jatra||*

'Sun God! Bless me with your rays so that my ears ring with celestial music and the effects of my past-life Karmas are washed away. Give us the physical and mental health to attain Moksha.'

*Hridrogamama Surya Harinanam Cha Nashanam|*

The Sun Salutation is good for the heart. The regular performer will live long, be hale and hearty, with a strong and a sturdy body and keen intellect.

**Offering Salutation to the Sun**
The first step consists of reciting the Sloka:
*Hiranmayena Patrena Satya Syapihitam Mukham|*
*Talvam Poshan Apa Vrunu satya Dharmayadrishtaye||*
'Oh Sun God! Your golden rays cover the door of Truth. Please open the door for this seeker of Satya (Truth) and Dharma (what is right).'

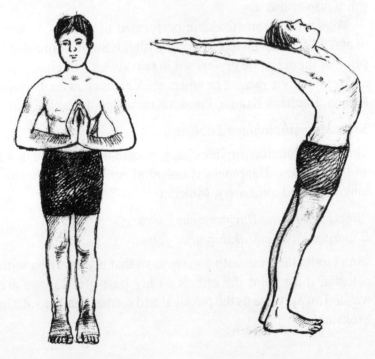

**Position of Sun Salutation**     **The Raised Arm Position**

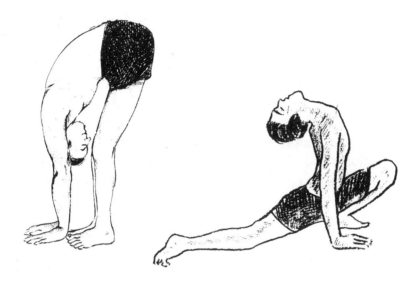

**The Hand to Foot Position**    **The Equestrian Position**

The next step in the Sun Salutation is to recite a set of mantras as listed below, breathing in deeply and then exhaling, in the standing posture for the salutation, which is known as the position of Samasthiti. The picture illustrates how it should be done. The mantras are:

1. *Om! Hram, Mitraya Nama:|*
2. *Om! Hrim, Ravayo Nama:|*
3. *Om! Hsim, Suryaya Nama:|*
4. *Om! Hreye Bhanave Nama:|*
5. *Om! Hraum, Khagaya Nama:|*
6. *Om! Hra, Pushne Nama:|*
7. *Om! Hram, Hiranya Garbhayanam:|*
8. *Om! Hrim, Mareechaye Nama:|*
9. *Om! Hrum, Aadhityaya Nama:|*
10. *Om! Hraimo, Savitre Nama:|*
11. *Om! Hraum, Arkaya Nama:|*
12. *Om! Hra, Bhaskaraya Nama:||*

With the last mantra, the hands, which were folded, are straightened, and air should be exhaled through the nose. This is followed by inhaling deeply while bending the body backwards as far as it will go, with the arms extended in line with the head as far as possible, as shown in the Raised Arm Position. The head is bent back until the forearms are seen.

This position is followed by moving in to the Equestrian Position smoothly. Puraka (inhaling) is done as the body straightens into a normal upright stand. Then do a Rechaka (exhaling), while moving to the intermediate Hand to Foot Position, before the Equestrian. As the legs are extended backwards for the Equestrian, the hands on the floor provide support. Then the chest is thrust forward, the head raised and the waist bent. The hands must be kept straight though, and the forelegs must not touch the floor. After this is completed, revert to a normal stand.

Now, after a Rechaka, it is time for the fifth posture of the Surya Namaskara, to put the knees on the floor, lifting the waist and contracting the abdomen, while the head is bent till one can see the umbilicus.

Thereafter, it is back to the Hand to Foot Position, with a Puraka (the sixth posture) followed by straightening (the seventh), and on to the Raised Arm Position, before concluding the Surya Namaskara by reverting to a normal standing position.

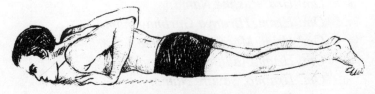

**The Eight-Limbed Position**

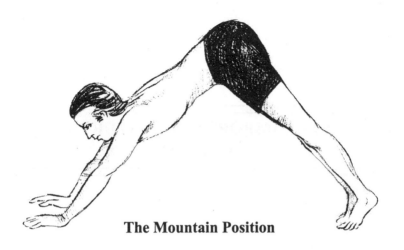

**The Mountain Position**

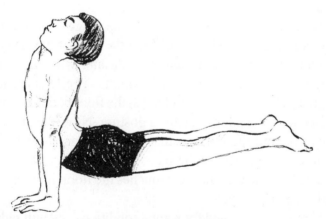

**The Cobra Position**

# 56

# SOME IMPORTANT POSTURES (ASANAS)

Asana is the word used for the postures which are intrinsic to the practise of Yoga. This chapter will deal with twenty-one basic Asanas which one needs to practise.

**Kurmasana**

The Kurmasana consists of the first six stages of the Surya Namaskara, followed by a Puraka at the start of the seventh, and then moving into a Bhuja Peedasana with the hands straight, placed between the thigh joints. The legs are then straightened. The cheek should touch the floor before the head is raised and one adopts a sitting posture. Now, the arms are brought behind the back so that the forefingers touch. The straightened legs should be placed one on top of the other while bending so that the head touches the floor, inhaling and exhaling on each cycle.

This exercise is good for Kapha conditions and will reduce the formation of phlegm in the chest and throat. It is also beneficial for the heart, lungs and the cardiovascular system, besides strengthening the chest and the back. Sufferers of angina pectoris (pain in the heart muscles) will find considerable relief should they practise this.

## Padmasana

This famous posture, known as the lotus position and universally used as illustration for texts on Yoga, is the classic posture for meditation. Lending itself to concentration, it improves the consciousness and the intellect, and brings about mental stability. On the physical level, it will reduce the fat in the thighs.

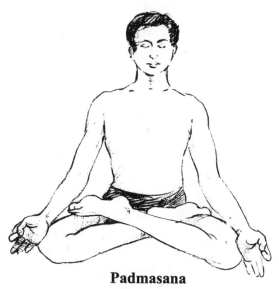

**Padmasana**

While sitting on the floor, bend the right knee first, so that the right foot is placed on the left thigh. Follow up similarly with the left knee so that the left foot is placed on the right thigh. Feet should be elevated, they must not touch the floor and so should the joints stay off the floor.

## Sarvangasana

This exercise stimulates the thyroid glands and the genitalia of both males and females. It is also useful in conditions of haemorrhoids, hernias and menstrual disorders.

**Caution:**

It is not to be practiced by people suffering from cervical spondylitis.

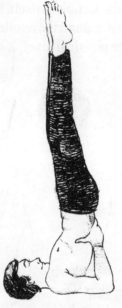

**Sarvangasana**

Lie down on a bed or the floor with the legs straight and the feet touching each other. Meanwhile, keep arms below the head and raise both legs together, swinging them smoothly till they are perpendicular to the bed, without bending the knees. Now bring the arms into play at the waist, raising the waist and the back with the help of the arms. The upper arms are kept firmly on the bed while the hands hold the back.

Having held this position, swing the legs gently towards the head, to be as close to parallel to the level of the bed as possible. With the support of the shoulders, heave upwards and hold the position for a period of two minutes, without shaking. Only the shoulder, the back of the neck and the back of the head should be touching the floor or the surface on which one is lying. The Asana ends by very slowly and carefully reverting to the normal prone position.

This exercise can also be performed as a variation when the stand is held for short bursts of five to eight seconds duration while breathing in and out.

## Matsyasana

This Asana is usually performed as a sequel to the Padmasana with which it acts as synergiser. In itself, it provides benefits to sufferers of bronchial asthma and Diabetes Mellitus.

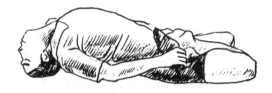

The Asana may be practiced in two styles, either sitting or lying.

Starting from a sitting position on the floor, move into the Padmasana posture. Then, the body is tilted backwards, with fingers interlocked behind the head and arms on the floor. Keeping hands on the floor, arch the back and neck into a bow shape so that the head and chest are off the floor. Once balanced in this state, catch the great toe of each foot with the index finger. Maintain posture for between half and a full minute before reverting to normal (*Samasthiti*).

The other way is to lie down on the back, with face up, before folding the legs so that the left foot is on the right thigh and vice versa. Then, bring the hands to the head before arching and follow the steps given above.

## Bhujangasana

This exercise is good for developing the ligaments of the back and beneficial for the sufferers of backache. It also benefits those with cough and respiratory disease, besides ridding the body of fat or adipose tissue around the abdomen.

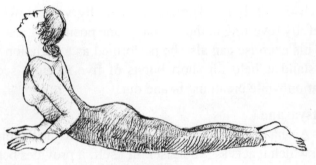

**Bhujangasana**

Lie down facing downwards, with legs extended and feet touching the ground. The face itself should be off the floor. Move arms forward by the side of the head and place palms on the ground. Then, move arms so that the palms which are flat on the ground reach the lower part of the rib-cage. Raise the head and upper torso by pushing downward till the elbows are in contact with the body. The back should form a semi-circle and extend the head as far as it will go. This has been likened to the posture of a snake. Thereafter, revert to normal.

**Dhanurasana**

An exercise that is meant for the relief of stomach disorders and to improve digestion, it is performed by lying face downwards on a surface, then bending the knee to catch the feet with each hand. The head and chest are then raised to make the body resemble an arrow.

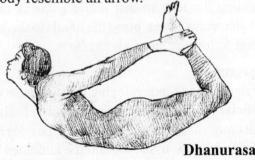

**Dhanurasana**

Look upwards while the entire weight of the body falls on the abdomen. Elbows must not flex. The position should be held briefly before reverting.

### Shirsasana

This exercise, which culminates in a headstand, enhances blood supply to the brain, besides providing a high level of conditioning to the body. It stimulates the thyroid and pituitary glands and is good for relieving a condition known as orchitis, as well as dysfunction connected with virility (disorders involving semen). It enhances blood flow to the brain and so benefits all brain functions.

### Caution:

It is not to be practised by people suffering from high blood pressure, otitis media (an affliction of the ear, which affects balance) and eye diseases.

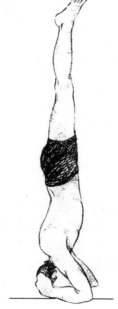

**Shirsasana**

Before starting the exercise, it is advisable to provide for some padding for the headstand, such as a bed-sheet or blanket folded three or four times over. Kneel on this padding, then bend over and place the elbows on the pad. The fingers should be interlocked while the elbows take a triangular placement, a tripod for balance.

The head is then cushioned in the hands. With the toes on the floor, the area between the knees and the waist is first raised, and then, the legs are raised till they are perpendicular to the ground. Hold this position for a while before reverting to normal.

## Shavasana

The simplest of postures, Shavasana, is the posture of tranquility. Good for relieving alleviated levels of blood pressure, inducing sleep and maintaining a tranquil state of mind, and creating a sense of peace.

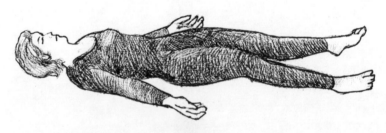

**Shavasana**

Simply lie down on a surface with the face upwards, arms relaxed and spread by the side. Every limb, including the legs, is kept loose and slightly spread. In this posture, try focussing the mind while the body is at complete rest.

## Vajrasana

This is another posture for meditation, but in addition it provides the benefits of relieving stiffness in the knees and legs and in relieving oedema.

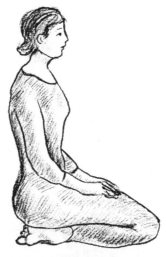

**Vajrasana**

The buttocks rest on the lower part of the legs and the feet, while the rest of the torso is straight. Palms rest on the thighs near the knees. Having achieved this position, bend from the waist and neck so that the head touches the floor. For meditation, keep the torso upright and close the eyes. Hold for as long as it suits the purpose.

## Hansasana

Primarily meant for the digestive system where it improves digestion, relieves constipation and stimulates the pancreas, this exercise helps the wrist joints to relax and strengthens the arms.

Bring the knees together with legs straight. Sit with the torso and the spinal column absolutely straight. Though similar to the Vajrasana, here, the hands are brought to the side of the waist. Then, part the knees and bend forwards till the elbows can rest on the floor. The weight of the body must be on the umbilical region, and the arms are bent to rest there. The head is then bent forward to touch the floor. Thereafter, the neck is raised so that one is facing fully forward. The body is in the shape of a "Z". Hold for a while before reverting to normal.

## Mayurasana
Another excellent exercise for the region of the abdomen, this promotes abdominal secretions, relieves indigestion and digestive disorders and conditions the muscles of the abdomen.

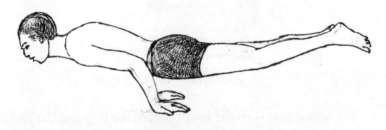

**Mayurasana**

Having adopted the first three stages of the Hansasana, the body is raised so that it is parallel to the floor, with just the arms for support and palms flat on the floor. The head is then raised, so that it faces forward. The arms are rotated and bent to come to a normal posture.

## Pavanamuktasana
An easier exercise for relieving constipation and digestive complications, this asana involves two stages.

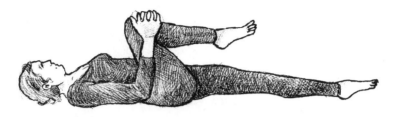

**Pavanamuktasana**

The first, called '*Ekapada Pavana Muktasana*', involves lying down in the relaxed style of the Shavasana before bringing the hands to the back of the head, breathing in deeply and raising the right leg to an angle of forty-five degrees, while the left leg is firmly on the floor. Then, while breathing in, the right leg is raised until perpendicular. Exhalation follows, accompanied by bringing of the knees towards the face, thigh to chest, and grasping the calves with the hands. Breathe in and out, raise and lower head for five times before repeating with the other leg.

The next stage is called '*Dwipada Pavana Muktasana*' and involves bringing both legs together, raising them to an angle of forty-five degrees without bending the knees. Next, while breathing in deeply, raising them so that they are perpendicular. Then, it is knee to chest, press and exhale. The chin is now brought up and the body twisted, first to the right so that the right arm touches the floor, and then, similarly to the left. This is repeated five times before reverting to normal.

**Supta Vajrasana**

A stimulant for the wrists, back and thighs, this posture brings relief to stiffness and pain in the back and the joints.

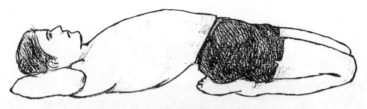

**Supta Vajrasana**

It starts with the legs and arms extended while lying on one's back. Then, the legs are bent from the knees so that the feet are next to and on the outer side of the hip. Forearms are then scissored under the head. Finally, the torso is raised from this position.

**Paschimottasana**

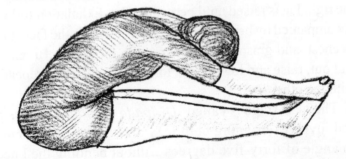

**Paschimottasana**

Lying down with legs extended, raise the hands to the ears. Then, breathing in and out deeply, raise the upper torso until it is perpendicular to the ground. While breathing out, bend forward, to catch the big toe with the index finger, keeping the face between the two knees and the forearms on the ground. Relax the muscles of the abdomen and the knees, and while holding position, breathe in and out, deeply, two or three times. Then, breathe in and raise the torso to return to normal.

## Chakrasana

This serves to stimulate the nervous system, and also provides benefits for conditions of asthma, constipation and diabetes.

## Caution:

It is not to be practiced by people suffering from stomach ulcers,slipped discs and heart disease.

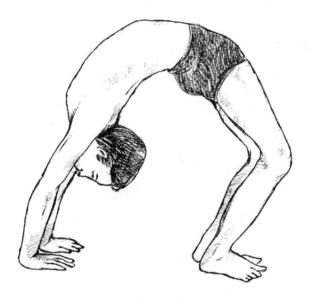

**Chakrasana**

Starting with lying on the back, the palms are placed flat on the floor and the feet are brought up, while the body is raised-so that it arches. Breathe in while arching, hold the position for two minutes and then breathe out while reverting to the normal.

### Swasthikasana

Another posture adopted while meditating, this helps the lower limbs to shed fat while removing stiffness in them. It is also good for the stimulation of the circulatory system and the mind.

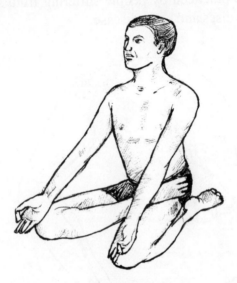

**Swasthikasana**

Sitting on the haunches, the right leg is bent so the right foot rests on the left thigh. Arms are extended, palms facing out, forefingers curled to touch the thumb – the Chinmudra Avastha. The position should be held for a minute or two or for the duration of meditation and prayer. Breathe in as the right leg is moved when reverting to normal.

### Bhadrasana

A simple exercise which shapes the thighs, it is beneficial for the bladder and the genito-urinary system.

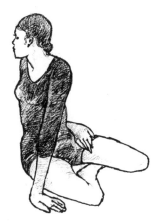

**Bhadrasana**

Sitting on the floor on one's haunches, legs bent at the knees, foot to hip, twist the torso to catch the toes with the fingers – the fingers of the right hand catching the left toes and vice versa. Hold position for a minute or two while breathing normally.

**Simhasana**

This is an exercise for the throat, the salivary glands and for sufferers of Tonsilitis.

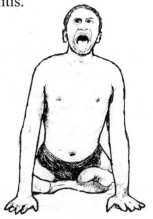

**Simhasana**

Assume the posture of the Padmasana. Then, push the body forward, its weight supported by the arms, fists clenched and on the floor. Stretch the neck out, extend the tongue as far as it will go and roar (like a lion).

## Siddhasana

Another classic pose for meditation, it was adopted by multitudes of sages over the years.

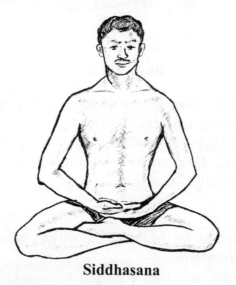

**Siddhasana**

Sit on the floor with knees apart and bent so that the calves touch the thighs. Keep the torso vertical and straight. Arms are brought to below the umbilicus and kept palm on palm. Breathe freely.

## Kukkutasana

An exercise that is good for relieving the Tridoshas, this helps those suffering from constipation and retention of urine. It works on the intestines and to trim the region around the pelvis.

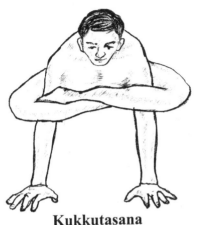

**Kukkutasana**

After assuming the Padmasana posture, push both hands between the folded legs down to the floor. Place the palms flat on the ground and push upward with the arms so that the body and the folded legs lift off the floor. The posture should be held for between one and three minutes before reverting to normal.

**Veerasana**
Lying flat on the ground, the right leg is brought to the left hip and the left leg is then bent back to bring the left heel to the thigh. Place hands on respective heels.

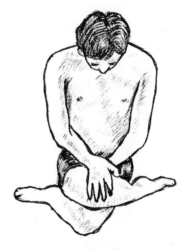

**Veerasana**

## Gomukhasana

This exercise is beneficial for the spinal cord, in treatment for abdominal disease and it aids in digestion.

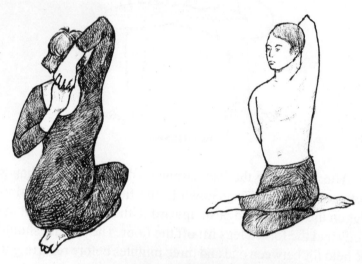

**Gomukhasana**

Sitting on a padded floor, bend legs keeping the right on the left, heels to the side of the left hip. With the torso vertical, raise the right arm, bend it behind the back while moving the left arm behind the back to lace the fingers of both hands.

# 57

# BREATH CONTROL
# (PRANAYAMA)

Prana is the Sanskrit word for life-force. Pranayama, then, is the term for practices which enhance life-force in people. Quite evidently, there must be a multitude of such practices and this has been the subject of debate among the sages and Yogis over the millennia. Shankara Bhagavatar put the number in thousands, while Swatmarama focused on just eight.

However,

*Surya Bhedena Mujjayi Seetkari Seetali Tatha|*
*Bha Streeta Bhramari Murcha Plavanityashtu Kumbhaka||*

Practising just four Pranayamas is sufficient for deriving health benefits for the body and the mind.

This is even more so when the individual practises the Pranayamas in conjunction with the exercises of Yoga, as the Geeta opines –

*Purvabhyasena Tenaivahriyate Hravashopisa:|*
*Asantasyakuta: Sukham|*

Without peace a man cannot be happy.

*Chalevate Chalam Chittam Nischale Nischalam Bhavet|*

Practise of Pranayamas with proper guidance helps a person achieve peace and develops his mind beyond the trivial.

*Yathashimhogaje Vyaghra: Bavedvashya: Sanai Sanai:|*
*Anyathahanti Sadhakam:||*

The power and skill over the lion and the tiger, that are demonstrated while capturing them, have to be replaced with patience and repetition in order to tame them. Applying this parable to the human body, the Vata may be controlled only through practise.

*Nyayatma Bala Hinena Labhya:|*
*Samedha Yana Bahunasrutena||*

A person with weakness of the senses will never attain anything. Mental strength and control over the senses is required to experience the spirit. Tranquility, peace and knowledge that are preventives of disease, poverty and unhappiness derive from repeated and regular practise.

**The four Pranayamas** consist of sets of breathing exercises for regulating the flow of *Pranavayu* (the breeze of life or the life-supporting part of air). To draw upon the example of weight-lifting, before lifting a heavy weight, we tend to breathe in, deeply. While lifting we hold our breath and exhale once the weight is lifted. Such regulation of breath is what Pranayama is about. The terms used are *Puraka* (inhaling), *Rechaka* (exhaling) and *Kumbhaka* (holding the breath).

**Puraka Pranayama** is to practise inhaling. This involves many forms of breathing – deep and shallow, emptying the lungs completely and then deep breathing, and controlling airflow inside the body. By properly practising this, it is possible to direct the air till it reaches the umbilicus.

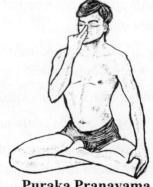

**Puraka Pranayama**

**Rechaka Pranayama,** also called *Bahyavritti Pranayama* by Patanjali, is the systematic practise of forms of exhaling. It involves a variety of techniques of breathing out from the nose and mouth, after holding one's breath for a while and circulating air through the lungs, the umbilicus, the heart, the throat and the nose.

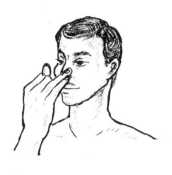

**Rechaka Pranayama**

**Kumbhaka Pranayama,** also called *Sthambhavritti Pranayama* by Patanjali, is the art of holding air inside of one. It involves the capability of holding the breath for long periods and utilising airflow within the body.

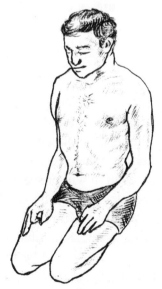

**Kumbhaka Pranayama**

**Abhyantara Pranayama** is performing a combination of the three Pranayamas. It develops from experience and individual practise varies depending on Desha, Kala and Sankhya (location and time). Normally, while performing a Abhyantara, the ratio between Puraka: Kumbhaka: Rechaka should be 1: 4: 2. This means, if breathing in is for 5 seconds, then breath must be held for exactly 20 seconds and exhaling must take exactly 10 seconds.

On the basis of time, Kumbhaka Pranayama is further classified into three types –
   a)  **Avar (Inferior):** In this, *Puraka* is of 8 seconds, *Kumbhaka* of 32 seconds, and *Rechaka* of 16 seconds.
   b)  **Madhyama (Medium):** In this, *Puraka* is of 16 seconds, *Kumbhaka* of 64 seconds, and *Rechaka* of 32 seconds.
   c)  **Pravar (Superior):** In this, *Puraka* is of 32 seconds, *Kumbhaka* of 128 seconds, and *Rechaka* of 64 seconds.

**Sudation by Pranayama:** For this purpose, after acquiring a comfortable sitting posture, one should close the right nostril and should breathe in to fill the lungs through the left nostril. *Kumbhaka* is done for a long time – until the face becomes red. Now, the left nostril is closed and breathing out is done through the right nostril. This is called *Agni Pradeepta Pranayama* or the Pranayama that ignites body fire and results in sweating or sudation. This should never be performed early in the practise. It should be practised daily and the duration of Kumbhaka should be increased gradually. It is capable of bringing on a sweat even in winter season.

Puraka and Rechaka should be done slowly without producing sound. Intensity of Kumbhaka should be increased gradually. In the first week, Kumbhaka should be of few seconds. In second week, it should be for eight seconds. In this way it should gradually be raised to sixty-four seconds.

When Abhyantara Pranayama is done to a ratio, it is known as *Sagarbha Pranayama*. If it does not follow a fixed ratio, it is known as *Nirgabha Pranayama*.

## The Rituals of Pranayama

1. It is customary for practitioners of Pranayama to perform it twice a day.
2. Before sunrise in the morning and after sunset in the evening are the best times.
3. It must be performed only in clean environs.
4. Fresh air should be plentiful.
5. It is performed when in either of three postures – Siddhasana, Padmasana or Vajrasana.
6. The posture should be practiced till one is comfortable in adopting it for durations of half an hour.
7. One should have previously practised the three *Bandhas*.

The Bandhas consist of Mula Bandha, Uddhiyana Bandha and Jalandhara Bandha. These are sub-routines – Mula Bandha is to sit in an Asana, then lift the anus and squeeze the flatus, while Jalandhara Bandha is to constrict and contort the throat muscles. They are explored in greater detail, in a later chapter.

## Forms of Kumbhaka Pranayama

*Surya Bhedanamujjayni Seetkaree Seetali Tatha|*
*Bastrika Brahmhari Murcha Plavinee Tyashta Kumbka Ka||*

... *{Hatha Yoga Pradeepika}*

The eight types of Kumbhka are -

1. Suryabhedana
2. Ujjayani
3. Seetkari
4. Seetali
5. Bastrika
6. Brahmhari
7. Murcha
8. Plavinee

## Suryabhedana Kumbhaka

*Asane Sukhade Yogi Buddha Va Chaivasanam Tata:|*
*Daksha Nadyam Samakrushy Bahistha: Pavanam Shanai:||*
*Akesha Dankha-graccha Nirodhavadhi Kumbhayet Tata:|*
*Shani: Sa Vyanadya Rechayet Pavanam Shanai:|*
*Kapala ShodhanamVata Doshaghnam Krimidosha Hrit|*
*Puna: Punaridham Karyam Surya Bhedana Muttaman||*
*... {Hatha Yoga Pradeepika}*

Sit in the Padmasana pose. Breathe in through the right nostril and hold your breath for some time. Then release breath (breathe out) slowly. This will relieve accumulation of Vata Doshas and act on worms and bacteria. It will also purify the mind.

## Ujjayani Kumbhaka Pranayama

*Mukhamsamyamya Nadebhyama Krusha Pavanamshanai:|*
*Yathalagathi Kantattu Hridayavadhi Saswanam|*
*Puvavat Kumbhayet Pranam Rechayedeedya Tata:|*
*Sleshmadoshaharam Kante Deharalavi Vardhanam*
*gacchatatishtata Karya Mujnaya Khyamtu Kumbhakam||*
*... {Hatha Yoga Pradeepika}*

Sit in the Padmasana pose. Breathe in as deeply as possible, through both nostrils (*Nasaputas*) and hold breath. Then release it through the left nostril. This will help alleviate Kapha, improve digestive fires, bring relief for nervous disorders and ascitis, and pacify disorders involving tissues (Dhatus).

## Seetkari Kumbhaka Pranayama

*Seet Takam Karaga Kuryat Tatha Vaktra Ghranenaiva*
*Vijrumbhakam|*
*Evamkhya Bhyasa Yogena Kama Deva Dwiteyaka:||*
*Yoginee Chakra Samanya Srusti Samhara Karaka:|*
*Nakshuddha Natrusha Nidra Naivalashyam Prajayate||*

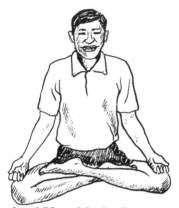

**Seetkari Kumbhaka Pranayama**

*Bhavet Satvam Chadehasya Sarvopadrava Varijita:|*
*Anema Vidhi Nasatyam Yogindra Bhumi Mandale||*
*... {Hatha Yoga Pradeepika}*

Sit in the Padmasana pose. Breathe out through both nostrils. Then fold the tongue backwards and press its tip to both the sides of the inner throat. Meanwhile, open the mouth slightly and make a hissing sound. Then, breathe in and hold breath for a while before releasing it through both nostrils. Continue repetitions for between one and five minutes.

**Seetali Kumbhaka Pranayama**

*Jihvaya Vayu Makrushya Purvat*
*Kumbha Sadhanam| Shankai*
*Ghrana Andhrabhyam Rechayet*
*Pavanam Sudhee:||*
*Gulma Pleehadikan Rogan*
*Jwaram Pittam Kshudha*
*Thrisham|*
*Vishani Seetali Nam Kumbhi*
*Keyam Nihanti Hi||*
*...{Hatha Yoga Pradeepika}*

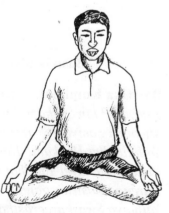

**Seetali Kumbhaka Pranayama**

Stick the tongue out slightly while curling it so the sides go upwards. Pressure from the lips makes it shaped like a narrowed canula tube. Breathe in gradually and hold breath before releasing. Repeat ten or twelve times. This procedure serves as treatment for –

1. Gulma (Fantom Tumours)
2. Enlargement of the spleen
3. Fevers
4. Bilious disorders
5. Appetite
6. Thirst
7. Cases of poisoning

It will relieve both the disease and its symptoms.

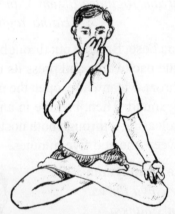

**Bastrika Kumbhaka Pranayama**

## Bastrika Kumbhaka Pranayama

*Samyak Padmasanam Baddhava Samgri Vodarasudhe:|*
*Mukham Samyamya Yatnena Pranam Ghranenarechyet||*
*Yathalaghat Hritkante Kapalavadhi Marutam|*
*Punarvirechayet Taddhat Purayecha Pun: Yathaiva Lauha*
*Karena Bhastravegana Chalyate|*
*Yathaiva Swashareerastham Chalaset Pavanamdhiya||*
*Yadasra Yo Bhaveddhe Tada Suryena Purayet||*

*Yathodaram Bhavet Purnam Anilena Tatha Laghu:||*
*Dharayet Nasikam Madhyatarjani Bhyam Venadrudham|*
*Vidhivat Kumbhakam Krutvarecha Yedeedyanilan*
*Kundalee Bodhakam Kshipram Pavanam Sukhamhitam|*
*Bahya Nadee Mukha Samsthaka Phadyargal Nashanam||*
*Visheshenaiva Kartavyambha Strakhyam*
*Kumbhakamidam||*

Breathe in and out, deeply and rapidly till exhausted. Then, take in air through the Suryanadi, close the Chandranadi and hold breath while closing the nostrils, using the thumb, the index and the last finger. Exhale through the Chandranadi and repeat for between one and five minutes. This will –
1. Stimulate the spinal cord
2. Alleviate the Tridoshas
3. Activate the Kundalini

## Brahmhari Kumbhaka Pranayama
*Vegad Ghosham Puraka Bringanadam Rechakammand Mandam|*
*Yogeendranameva Manyasa Yogatchitte Jataka Chidananda Leela||*

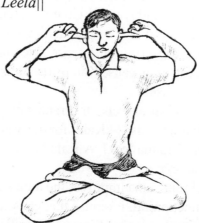

**Brahmhari Kumbhaka Pranayama**

After assuming the illustrated posture, perform a sound Bringanad through both nostrils and hold breath. Then make a buzzing sound and exhale gradually. This stimulates the brain, provides a sense of bliss, is good for the ligaments, improves voice and produces pleasantness in the mind.

## Murcha Pranayama

*Anta: Pravartitodara Maruta Puritodara:| Payasyagadhepi Sukhan Plavate Padma Putravat|*

Take a deep breath and expand the stomach before a gradual exhalation. It creates a feeling of lightness.

## Plavinee Pranayama

Puraka Pranayama may create a bloating of the stomach which should be relieved by exhaling to remove air. It is a good exercise for mental calm and moves the mind towards Samadhi.

**Siddhanta** is the term for custom and although it dictated that Pranayama be performed four times a day at intervals of six hours, a frequency of twice or thrice a day is adequate. There are three levels at which Pranayama may be performed. These are Pravara, Madhya and Uttama. Uttama stands for ultimate and practise at levels approaching the Uttama, such as the Kanishka, can bring on intense sweating. Practise at the Uttam level can often cause Kampa (tremors and shaking). If so, stop the exercise.

The duration of an exercise in Pranayama is fixed at 12 Kalas for the Avara levels, 24 Kalas for the Madhya level and 36 Kalas for the Uttama level. A Kala is the time it takes to shut and open an eye.

Eventually, Pranayama improves the lung's and the heart's capacities of functioning. Exercise that causes sweating and palpitations before beginning the practise will scarcely affect the practitioner later. Coupled with Yoga, tremendous increase in one's vital capacity can be achieved.

A yardstick that may be used is that healthy people respire at the rate of sixteen to eighteen times a minute. Sweating may also be an indicator of health. It was said–

*Sramanasweda Jalpadhyam Sm Vinmurcha Jayet Yada||*
Sweda or sweat is a sign of fatigue setting in, so the weak will break into a sweat, with even moderate exertion. With proper practise of Pranayama, one gradually overcomes the tendencies of sweating or feeling faint when exerting. Also, the skin is the seat of the Vata and sweating overmuch is not good for its tone and condition. By pacing one's Pranayama, sweating can be avoided. Levels at which one performs should be raised gradually. Accordingly, *"Jalenasrama Jatenagatra Mardana Macheret| Drudhata, Laghuta Chaivatene Gatrasya Jayate||"*

A diet that is rich in dairy products like milk and ghee is good for practitioners, especially in the starting phase. Those who are accustomed to Pranayama on the other hand, require no special diets. For them, normal, routine fare will be sufficient.

The **Hatha Yoga Pradeepika** is an ancient text, which is considered to be a classic on Yoga and related practices. Some of its comments about Pranayama are:

*Ayuktabhyasa Yogena Sarvaroga Samudbhava:*

Pranayama has the capability of curing all diseases, if practiced properly.

*Hikkaswasascha Kasascha Sira: Karnakshi Vedhana Prakopata:||*

Improper practice of Pranayama can produce diseases of the Vata in the region of the head. Ailments such as *Hikka, Swasa* (dyspnoea) and *Kasa* (coughing), and problems with the *Akshi* (eyes) and *Karna* (ears), brought about because of vitiation of Pranavayu. Aberrations and contraction will occur in the *Spotas* (channels and passages) leading to ailments.

*Yuktam Yuktam Trajet Vayum: Yuktam Yuktam Cha Purayet|*
*Yuktam Yuktam Cha Vadhniyat: Evam Siddham Va Puryat||*
Practice of the components of Pranayama – Puraka, Rechaka and Kumbhaka – is a gradual process. Starting slowly, but progressing steadily. Done properly, the purification of the Ida, the Pingla and the Nadi Chakras will take place. This will create awareness in the Kundalini followed by Sasrara. This results in the state of Siddhavastha. These concepts are explored later.

252

# 58

# CLEANING INTERNAL TRACTS AND FACETS OF YOGA (SHATKARMA AND SAMADHI)

The Human Body consists of organs, tissues and cells composed of molecules of matter. In addition to these material constituents, which in the terminology of Ayurveda are called Doshas, Dhatus and Malas, there is the mind. The mind is less tangible than the body but its functioning is apparent, and together, the body and the mind make up the human being. The subtle and less tangible components that go to make the mind are the Atma, Indriyas and the Manas. The term that Ayurveda and Yoga use for these constituents is *Ghataka*. The material ones, which make up the bo ly, are known as *Sthula Ghataka,* while the ethereal, which make up the mind, are known as the *Sukshma Ghataka.* Both the kinds are interdependant and must themselves interact in harmony for the entire being to exist in a state of wellness.

Therapies, or *Karmas*, have been evolved in Ayurveda and Yoga to rectify imbalances and maintain just such harmony. In Ayurveda, it is the Panchakarma Therapy after Purva Karma. In Yoga, it is a set of six therapies that are collectively called the *Shatkarmas.*

*Meda: Sleshmadhika Purvam Shat Karmani Samacharet|*
*Anyastu Nacharothaam Doshanam Sama Bhavata:||*
                                        *... {Hatha Yoga Pradeepika}*

Adopting the Shatkarmas is the best method of treating an excess of fat and Kapha in the body. This is not required by the healthy.

*Dhautirvastishatha Neti Stratakam Naulikam Tatha|*
*Kapala Bhati Schaitani Shatkarmi Prachakshate||*

The six Shatkarmas are:
1. Dhauti
2. Vasti
3. Neti
4. Trataka
5. Nauli
6. Kapala Bhati

The mind must be properly prepared before these may be adopted.

**Dhauti Karma:** This consists of washing and flushing the alimentary tract (*Annavahasrotas*). The alimentary tract contains Pitta in the lower part of the stomach till the umbilicus, and Kapha all over. This treatment is meant for purifying both the Doshas. There are three different procedures for this therapy –
1. Vastra Dhauti
2. Kunjala or Gojakarani Dhauti
3. Danda Dhauti

**Vastra Dhauti:** The procedure has been detailed in the Hatha Yoga Pradeepika as follows–

*Chaturangula Vistaram Hastapancha Dhashayatam|*
*Gurupadishta Margena Siktam Vastram Shanai Graset|*
*Puna: Pratyahare Chetdu Dinatam Dhauti Karmatat||*

It involves swallowing a piece of cloth soaked in water and the steps are outlined below:
   i. A strip of cloth, which is 1 Angula wide and of 15 hands in length, is taken.

ii. This is washed thoroughly and sterilised in hot water.

iii. A few days are spent on practising how to swallow this strip. At first, just a little is swallowed, and gradually over the days, more and more, until one is relatively comfortable and the gag reflex has been somewhat overcome.

iv. Finally, the strip is swallowed almost completely, until just a bit remains outside the mouth. This serves as a tag to use in pulling the strip out, once the procedure has been concluded.

v. Prior to the swallowing, a litre of brine (common salt in hot water) must be drunk. It should be understood that one is likely to gag and throw up.

vi. As the Vastra or strip is pulled out, it will carry with it the vitiated Kapha. The process of removal should be slow and gradual.

As listed in the Hatha Yoga Pradeepika, the benefits are –

*Kasa Swasa Pleehya Kushtam Roga Scha Vimshati||*

a) Curing a cough

b) Curing Dyspnoea

c) Normalising an enlarged spleen

d) Curing diseases of 20 kushtas

**Kunjala Dhauti:** This stands for induced vomiting, and other synonymous terms for it are *Gajakarani Dhauti* and *Vamana Dhauti*. Vomiting may be induced in any way, whether by drinking large quantities of very salty water, or by inserting a finger and tickling the throat. While throwing up, as the stomach churns and twists, it must be ensured that the body is bent at ninety degrees from the waist.

Commonly employed to remove ingested poison, it benefits cases of indigestion, some skin conditions and rheumatoid arthritis.

**Caution:**
It is not to be practised by people with heart disease.

**Danda Dhauti:** This combines the other two. Here, vomiting is induced by swallowing or inserting a cloth or rubber strip. An additional precaution is taken of knotting the part that will stay outside the mouth so that it is not swallowed accidentally. Before insertion, the cloth or rubber strip should be washed with hot water three or four times and salt water drunk until the stomach is full. It takes about seven minutes to perform, till the contents of the stomach come out. Its benefits are -

(a) Curing diseases of the Kapha and the Pitta
(b) Relieving flatulence
(c) Relief from the effects of bronchial asthma
(d) Control over the swings in sugar level in case of Diabetes Mellitus

Dhauti may be combined with Nauli Karma, which is detailed below, by regular practitioners of Yoga.

**Nauli Karma**

*Amandavarta Vagena Tudam Samvya Pasam Vrita:|*
*Natam-sobramaye Deshanauli: Sidhe:Prachakshate||*

By moving and exercising the ligaments and muscles of the stomach, it is possible to work on the alimentary tract. This definitely requires practise. Contorting the stomach to the right side is called *Dakshana Nauli,* while contorting it to the left constitutes *Vama Nauli.*

Before the actual Nauli procedure, preparation by way of Udiyana Bandhana and Agnisara Kriya is made. The Nauli begins by sitting on a stool, or in the Padmasana style on the floor. Now follow a Rechaka Pranayama and a Kumbhaka

Pranayama before focusing the inner faculties to conceiving the Nauli in the middle of Udara or the Madhya Nauli.

The benefits are –

(a) Pacification of the Doshas.

(b) Relief for the diseases of the Doshas.

(c) Increase in digestive fire.

(d) Proper digestion of food and assimilation of nutrients.

(e) Promotes à sense of well-being in the individual.

(f) Conditions the abdominal area.

(g) Cleanses the stomach.

(h) Removes constipation and facilitates bowel movement, thereby not allowing waste to accumulate.

Nauli, the controlled movement of the stomach and intestines, is a basic and important part of Yoga.

## Kapala Bhati

*Bhasthra Valloha Karasyarechs Purasa Sambhramau| Kapala Bhati Vrikhyata Kaphadosha Vishoshanee||*

*... {Hatha Yoga Pradeepika}*

This is performed while sitting in the Padmasana, with the spinal column absolutely straight. Then, a few Rechakas (exhalations) are done very quickly so that the muscles of the stomach are drawn in towards the vertebral column. The exhalation is followed by a slow release of the muscles of the stomach, while slowly breathing in. The pace is then increased from forty to a hundred and twenty times a minute.

After this, it will take a minute or so for the respiration to revert to normal. The benefits of this procedure are –

(a) Producing a tranquility of the mind

(b) Expelling built up carbon dioxide

(c) Stimulation of the cells of the body

(d)Purification of the respiratory channel

(e)Conditioning of the stomach muscles

## Nadishuddhi

*Yadatu Nadi Shuddhi: Syat Tada Chiharananibahtyata:||*
*Kayasya Krushata Kanti Sada Jayate Nischitam|*
*Yatheshta Dhaaran Vaayo Ranalasya Pradeepanam|*
*Nadabhivyakti Rarogyam Jayate Nadishodhanam||*

*... {Hatha Yoga Pradeepika}*

This exercise is meant for the purpose of purifying the nerves. The relaxed posture in a kneeling position is good for meditation. Note that the index finger of the right hand is pointed at the medula in the centre of the forehead and held there for a while. By acting on the nerves, this exercise is beneficial for many parts of the body and its functioning.

## Pratyahara

Yoga is Astanga, meaning that it is eight faceted. Pratyahara is the fifth of these eight facets. It seeks to enhance control over the Indriyas, the set of qualities or mental propensities that go to make up individual personality. Some references about it from the scriptures are produced below –

*Chitta Syantamurkhi Bhava Pratyahara|*

*... {Trishikhi Brahmnopishad}*

Man's aim in all activity is to be able to perceive the Brahma.

*Vishayebhya: Indriyarthebhyo Manonirodhanam*
*Pratyahara:|*

*... {Upanishad}*

With the practise of Pratyahara, one will cease being preoccupied with this world and move towards the Brahma.

*Yat Pashyatitutat Sarvam Cittasya Swarupanu Kara*
*Evendriganam Pratyahara:||*

*... {Patanjali's Yogadarshana}*

When the mind exerts control over propensities, it is an act of Pratyahara

*Tata Paramavasyatendriyanam|*

*... {Patanjali's Yogadarshana}*

To overcome succumbing to desires, one has to practise. Prayer and Vairagya help and are part of Pratyahara.

## Dharana

Conceptualisation and imagination are near equivalents for the concept of Dharana. It is one of three Sadhanas of Antaranga and application of Dharana shifts the personality from a state of Chitta (reactive, animalistic) to Chaitanya (capable of higher thought processes). In classical terms, Dharana meant concentrating one's mind on either a centre of the brain or on a devotee of God or on the Almighty Himself. Focussing on Surya, Chandra, Krishna or idols were tools used for Dharana and by using the Kapala (brain), qualities such as Dhee (intellect), Dhriti (steadfastness) and Smriti (memory) were developed.

## Dhyana (Meditation)

Meditation is a very important part of Yoga. The word *Dhyana* is derived from *Dhaichintay* which means to think deeply about a thing or subject. Through meditation, one attains Atmajnana or knowledge about the soul, and from this a vision about oneself and the world emerges with clarity and simplicity.

*Moksha: Karmakshayadeva Sa Chatma Jnana To Bhavet|*
*Dhyana Sadhyam Matam Tach Chatat Dhyanam Hita*
*Matman:||*

*... {Hatha Yoga Pradeepika}*

With meditation, man can recall experiences from past life as well as this one. By pondering over and learning from these, he will not be overly entangled with the happenings of this world. This is the state of Atmajnana. He will then submit himself to *Eswara* (God), the state of *Karmakshaya* and attain Moksha.

*Dhyanam Nirvisha Yammana|*

... *{Mandalopanishad}*

While animals are limited to only having **Chetana** (compulsive desires), all men have Atma, which should be allowed into meditation. Such thinking becomes Dhyana.

While the practice of meditation for sustaining health has been a principle followed in India for ages, the world has also been aware of this for some time now. Studies have been conducted on the emission of waves from the brain and effective techniques have been developed for meditation. These have been employed for a variety of purposes, ranging from treatment of stress to cures for cancers.

**Samadhi**
This is the eighth facet of Yoga, enabling the practitioner to reach a state from which salvation is possible. This is the ultimate objective of the practice of Yoga.

*Tadevartha Matra Nibhrámse Swarupa Shunyameva Samadhi:|*

... *{Yoga Darshana}*

Bring together the Dhyata, Dhyana and Dhyeya to merge with the cosmos, the stage of Samadhi.

*Yoga: Samadhi Samamyetyam Labdava Samadhi Prakeertita:|*

... *{Amruta Madopanishad}*

When the Atma (one's soul) combines with the Paramatma (the Eternal or Supreme Soul), or when the mind has discharged Chaitanya (has overcome all worldly desires), or when, with Dhyana, man is able to envision the Parmatma with his own Atma, then does he achieve Samadhi. All these states are Samadhi and even though the descriptions vary, they are one and the same. The person becomes a *Soham Brahma*, an extension of Brahma.

*Sarvarthatai Kagrasado Kshyodayao|*
*Chittasya Samadhi Parinam:||*

... *{Yogasutra, 11:3}*

Man's objective is to arrive at Samadhi, a state of continuous meditation and suspended animation. His motor and other senses are in a state of rest, similar to sleep. His Manas (mind) and his Buddhi (intellect), on the other hand are active and he will be able to visualise the creations of the world, Kama (sex) and his Karma (work) in the perspective of the Parmatama. Such a being will forsake all worldly affairs as he transports to the inner world of God and hears celestial music. In this state, he will perceive the past, present and future.

Samadhi can take two forms as described below.

### Samprajnata Samadhi

The mind develops habits or *Vrittis*. Vrittis include the simplest, such as a way of walking or eating meals, to the complex attachments that we form with the material world. Remaining bound to our Vrittis commits us to a cycle of rebirth and will not allow merger with the Cosmos. Samadhi achieved by spurning attachments to the *Bahyajat Jagat,* the material world, is called *Savikalpa* or Samprajnata *Samadhi.*

## Asamprajnata Samadhi

The purpose of Yoga was to develop a system of practise that would climax with the attainment of Moksha or salvation, a state when the mind fuses with God and the two merge into one. This act of fusion is called the *Visarjana* of *Samskara*. This is the *Charama Avastha* or the ultimate state of Yoga. It is the point of Samapti or conclusion, when the mind dissociates from the material world, all the *Kleshas* (afflictions) vanish along with Drishya (images), Drishta (sight) and Indriyaas (senses).

# 59

# CONCEPTS OF IDA AND PINGLA

The Head is called **Uttamanga** in the terminology of Yoga, literally the ultimate limb. It is the centre, the seat of all the activities of the mind and it functions through the *Naditantras*. *Nadi* is the term for ducts, veins and tubes, so the Naditantras make up the brain and the nervous system. Mental activity consists of *Chinta* (thinking), *Vichara* (judgement), *Ooha* (conjecture), *Dhyeya* (rationale) and *Sankalpa* (imagination). It is the system of Naditantras that permit these activities to be done in conjunction and in fact, to be at all individually performed. These activities occur with stimulation from the variety of **Indriyas** that go to constitute the mentality of each person. Indriya is the term for our mental faculties, such as perception and cognizance. Accordingly, we have a number of Indriyas and Ayurveda puts it at five Karmendriyas (the functional Indriyas) and five Jnanindriyas (the knowledge Indriyas, such as memory). Our individual Indriyas, along with Naditantra and Nadiyantra (mechanism) determine our personality. Control over these, mean control over the mind and this is the philosophy or dictum (Siddhanta) of Shadchakras and Kundalinis.

Ida and Pingla provide the connectivity between the Chakras. Ida stands for the energy in sympathetic nerves, while Pingla stands for the energy in parasympathetic nerves in the spinal column. Ida (or Eda), channelled through the Chandra

Nadi, and Pingla, channeled through the Surya Nadi, are located to the right and left side of the spinal cord respectively.

The Chakras are:

1. Muladhara Chakra – the pelvic plexus
2. Sarvadishtana Chakra – the interior mesentric plexus
3. Mani Puraka Chakra in the Nabhi – the epigastric plexus
4. Anahata Chakra in the heart – the cardiac plexus
5. Vishuddhakhya Chakra in the throat – the pharyngeal plexus
6. Ajna Chakra between the eyebrows – the medulla

*Sarvendriyani Cha|*
*Tadutta Manga Manganam Sirastadabhi Deeyatet||*

*... Charaka*

When Chittavritti is opposed, energy flows through the Sushma Nadi (spinal cord) to the Sahasra and the centre. Samadhi is achieved.

*Nadyesananta Samutpanna Sushumna Pancha Parvasu*

Nadis form on four sides of the spinal cord.

*Tata Urdwotalu Mule Sahsrara Sushobhinam|*
*Astiyara Sushumnaya: Mulam Savivaram Sthitam||*
*Talu Mule Sushumnasa Adhovaktra Pravartate| Muladharena*
*Yosnanta Sarvonadi Samasrita:||*

Refers to the brain stem (root of Talu in the head), the cells,spinal cord and cerebrospinal fluid. From the roots, the Nadis (nerves) go to the pelvic plexus.

*Edapingala Bhagavati Ganga Pingalayamu Na Nadee|*
*Edapingalayo Madhya Sushumna Cha Sarawatee||*

The system of Ida and Pingla has been likened to the river system where the Jamuna flows to its confluence with the

Ganga. Yoga releases the power in the Chakras for activity. This is the process of Mandalini.

*Vayu Stantra Yantradhara:*
The structures of the body are composed of Vata.

*Urdhwa Mula Madha: Shakha Mrushaya:|*
*Purushyam Vidu:|*
*Mula Praharina Stasmat Rogan Sheeghra Taram Jayet|*
*Sarvendriyani Ye Nasimin Prana: Yena Cha Samshrita:|*
*Tena Tashyotta Mangasyarakshyayaa Maadrute Bhavet|*
...{*Vagbhata*}

Inspiration springs from the interaction of the brain and the nerves. Through the Ida and the Pingla, this reaches out to every corner and extremity of the body. Treatment given to the body should in no way harm or injure the brain, as it is the seat of the Prana and the Indriyas.

# 60

# NASAL THERAPY
# (NAULI KARMA)

Nauli Karma can be of either the *Jala Neti* or the *Sutra Neti* kind. It is a process for periodically cleaning the internal area of the nose and mouth.

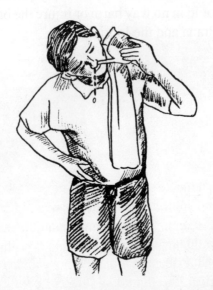

**Jala Neti**
Here, water is drawn through the nose until it fills the nasal passages and the mouth, before letting it out through the mouth. The equipment consists of a vessel with an attached

tube meant for insertion into one nostril. Water taken in through one nostril may also be expelled from the other. Either Ghee or milk or salt is added to the water used for this purpose.

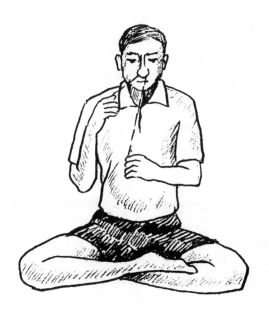

## Sutra Neti

A thread, which must be thick enough not to cut into the lining of the nose and mouth, preferably absorbent and about the length of one's arm, is taken and inserted into the nasal passage. It should be thoroughly cleaned in boiling water and smeared with a lubricant before insertion. Once its tip appears out of the mouth, the thread should be manipulated to and fro, for a thorough cleaning of the passages, after which it is removed by pulling it out of the mouth.

The following excerpts have been taken from the scriptures:

*Kapalashodhami Chaiva Divya Dushti Pradayani|*
*Urdhwajatrugatan Rogan Neti Rashu Nihanti Cha|*
*... {Hatha Yoga Pradeepika}*

*Vigata Ghananishotha Prataruthayanityam Pibatikhalu*
*Naroyo Bheemarandrenavari|*
*Nabhavati Mati Purna Schakshu Sha Tarkeshya Tullo*
*Balipalito Vihin: Sarva Rogai Virmukta:||*
*... {Acharya Bhavaprakash}*

Keeping water in a copper vessel overnight and drinking it in the morning is beneficial. It will provide the benefits of Ushapana.

*Arsha: Shotha Grahanyo Javara, Jatara Kushta, Medho*
*Vikara:|*
*Mutraghatasara Pitta Sravana Galasira:|*
*Sroni Sulaksha Roga:||*
*Yochanye Vata Pittaja Kapha Kruta Vyadhayoi: Santi*
*Jantho:||*

Nauli provides cures for the following diseases:

1. Haemorrhoids
2. Oedema
3. Sprue
4. Fevers
5. Stomach disease
6. Stricture of Urethra
7. Haemorrhagic Diathesis
8. Tonsilitis
9. Sinusitis

# 61

# FLUSHING THE INTESTINES
# (VASTI KARMA)

Employing Enema to flush the large intestine is called Vasti Karma. This is a procedure which is to be conducted sparingly because the large intestine happens to be the seat of the Vata and frequent flushing of this part will aggravate Vata. The fluid which is used for the enema can either be a decoction of herbs in water, in which case it is called *Niruha Vasti*, or an emulsion of oil and water, in which case it is called *Anuvasana Vasti*. Schedules for such therapy, which is administered in multiples of eight, need to be prepared with the guidance of an Ayurvedic doctor.

*Nabhidadhnajale Payau Nyasta Nalo Uktasana:|*
*Adhara Kunchanam Kuryat Kshalanam Vastikarmatat:||*
*... {Hatha Yoga Pradeepika}*

While in a tub in the Uktasana posture, send the water up the intestinal tract into the large intestines.

It may be applied while the receiver is in a sitting position in a tub, and the nozzle is smeared with oil, glycerine or ghee as lubricant. The water flushes the intestines and comes out with faecal matter and other doshas.

The benefits of Vasti are:

*Gulma Pleehodara Cha Pi Vata Pitta Kaphodbhava:|*
   It is part of the curing process for diseases such as –

1. Gulma (Fantom Tumours).
2. Pleehodara (Ascitis and enlargement of the spleen).
3. All diseases of Vata, Pitta and Kapha.

*Dhatveendriyanta: Karnam Prasadam Dadyacha Kanti Dahana Pradeeptim:||*

                                   ... *{Hatha Yoga Pradeepika}*

Its other benefits are -

1. It creates pleasantness in the senses.
2. It tones the skin.
3. It improves digestive fires.
4. It cleanses the gut and removes any excesses of all the three doshas that may be present there.

**Caution:**

It is not to be administered to people suffering from tuberculosis, sprue, inflammation of the intestines and the anus, severe dyspnoea and gastroenteric ailments like typhoid.

# 62

# EXERCISING THE EYES
# (TRATAKA)

Trataka is the term in Yoga for exercising the eyes and can be of three kinds – Bhaya, Madhya and Abhyantra.

**Bhaya Trataka** consists of simply exercising the eyes by focussing on distant objects in a panorama. By focussing on mountains, trees, the moon and so on. Of course, one should never look at the sun as it will damage the eyes. It improves the vision besides being useful for Vata Rogas, such as nervous diseases, and for Chandra Grahadoshas.

**Madhya Trataka** – Sitting Padmasana style in a comfortable and peaceful environment, one focuses the eyes on an object placed at eye level, less than two metres away. This object can be a candle or burning lamp, an "Om" written on a white piece of paper, a black dot on a wall or a figurine.

While the looking (gazing) is supposed to be intense, the exercise should be terminated once tears result. In addition to the benefits to vision, Madhya Trataka is a way of improving one's powers of concentration.

It is not recommended for those suffering from sexually transmitted disease, high blood pressure and retinal problems.

**Abhyantara Trataka** consists of focus on an object very close to the eyes, typically on the front part of the nose in between the eyebrows.

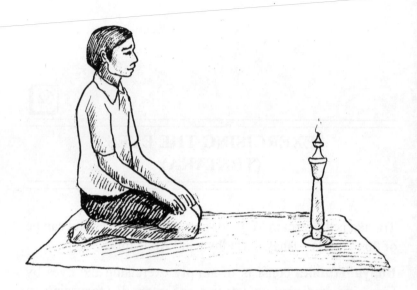

It is beneficial for those with a Pitta constitution and what
is called Hridayaa-bhimukhi. It is supposed to increase
compassion in the practitioner and will relieve burning
sensations in the heart, eyes and nose.

# 63

# SUB - ROUTINES
# (BANDHA)

Reference was made to the three **Bandhas** in an earlier chapter, in connection with the procedures of conducting Pranayama. The term 'sub-routine' was applied to the Bandhas because while they are not exercises in themselves, they involve exercise of internal organs and body parts in order to enhance the benefit of the exercise that they form a part of.

Pranayama is based on inhaling Pranavayu, and a sign of improved lung function is the capacity to hold one's breath longer and longer. Also, the more Pranavayu that we can take in the better it is. After all, it is Pranavayu (oxygen) that carries out every bodily activity. The object of Pranayama is to improve lung function.

The Bandhas make it possible for us to inhale more and deeper; just as our chest and abdominal area swell as we breathe in and subside as we breathe out, while when we hold our breath, the stomach, our anus and throat constrict.

## Jalandhara Bandha
*Kanta Kunchana Purvakam Chibukasya Hridi Sthapanam Jalandhara Bandha:|*

After breathing in (Puraka), the throat muscles are contracted, the chin is made to touch the chest, while holding air in the throat area. The uvula is contracted similar to when taking food.

### Mula Bandha

*Adha: Pradeshat Akunchanamiti Mulabandha:|*

Mulabandha is a contraction of the Muladhaara Chakra, the first of the Adhastachakras. While sitting in the Siddhasana posture with the left heel near the scrotum, contract the anus and lift the body. This awakens the Kundalini and activates the Manovaha Srotas.

### Uddiyana Bandha

*Prayatna Visheshena Nabhi Pradeshasya Prishtata:|*
*Akarshana Mudiyana Bandha:|*

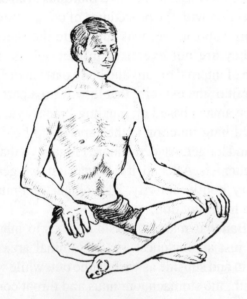

**Uddiyana Bandha**

The abdomen is drawn in and raised while breathing out. Air is completely exhaled when a full effort is made to squeeze the stomach muscles towards the vertebral column. This empties the body of all the used up air. The Kumbhaka that follows will have large quantities of fresh Pranavayu. This

Bandha should be practised with Kumbhaka as well. It will move the Prana through the subtle centres and obstruct its movement downwards.

# 64

# YOGA AND AYURVEDA AS RELIEVERS OF STRESS AND UNHAPPINESS

Moksha, or Salvation, is the final objective of the four stages of man, the Purushartha (raison d'être of adulthood). Yoga offers a path to final salvation as well as a more temporal kind, temporal in terms of relieving unhappiness, the kind that certainly results from poor health. We consist of the Sthula Ghatakas, the Doshas, Dhatus and Malas, combined with the Sukshma Ghatakas, the Atma, Indriyas and Manas. Yoga helps in balancing these properly. For the Yogi, though, some tenets are to be observed.

*Samutyam Yogaucchate|*

*Dosha Samyamarogata| Samyam Prakritruchyatet||*

Prajnaparadha is the main cause for all disease.

*Mana Evamanushyanam Karnam Bandha Mokshaya|*
*    ... {Charaka Samhita Shareerasthaana, Chapter 1}*

This text opines that Prajnaparadha will not be produced if one –

1. Does service for good people
2. Keeps good company and shuns bad company
3. Studies the Dharma Granthas (religious texts)
4. Observes fasts

5. Develops knowledge of the Adhyatma
6. Is without Ahamkara (arrogance)
7. Strives towards the Samadhi (fusion) of the Manas (personality) and Buddhi (intellect)

*Smritva Swabhavam Bhavanam Smaran Dukhat*
*Pramuchyate|*
    *... {Charaka Samhita Shareerasthana}*

With the awareness of one's Karmas (past actions) and unhappiness, if one strives, one will attain salvation. Both Ayurveda and Yoga promote health, and Ayurveda balances the Doshas, Dhatus and Malas. Rasayana (nutrition) must be given to people with bad precedents in past and present life.

*Atmendriya Manorthanam Sannikarshat Pravartate|*
*Sukhadukha Manaram Bhadhatma Sthemanasisthire|*
*Nivartate Tadubhayam Vaseetvam Chopajayayte|*
*Sa Shareeasya Yoga Jnastvam Yoga Mrushayo: Vidu:||*
    *... {Charaka Samhita Shareerasthana, 1:138, 139}*

Happiness and unhappiness are both derivatives of the Atma, Indriyas and Manas. If the body and its personality are under control, these can be directed to the path of happiness(*Chittavritti Nirodha*). In Yoga and salvation there is no pain.

*Yoga Moksha Cha Sarveshaam Vedananamavartanam|*
*Moksha Nivrithi Nishshesha: Yoga Moksha Pravarthaka:||*
    *... {Charaka Samhita Shareerasthana}*

Unhappiness (Dukha) is the product of Adhyatmika, Adibhoutika and Adhidaivika.

*Punarapi Jananam Punarapi Maranam|*
*Punarapi Jananee Jatare Shayanam|*

Man will be born and will die. In this world, man always thinks of his stomach (creature cravings). Always thinking about his happiness in this world, it would be better for him to focus his Manas and Atma to the Parmatma for peace, happiness and health. Yoga can help him in this search for salvation.

# 65

# RAJAYOGA AND HATHAYOGA

Yoga is a link to connect the soul (one's Atma) to God, the Super Soul (Parmatma). Yoga is a process by which the adult (Purusha) gives up animalistic cravings to create a connection with God. The Patanjali Yoga Sutra says –
*Yogash chitt vritti nirodha|*
Doing away with mundane and trivial desires arising in the mind is known as Yoga.

The Mind is an ocean of material desires, not only from the present life, but also from previous lives. The mind, along with the subtle body, a term for the senses and the soul together (which constitute *Ayu*), transmigrates from one body to another. Desires, many of which are either mundane or unhealthy, are embedded in the subconscious memory and keep arising in the mind. These preoccupy the mind to the extent that higher conceptualisation is impossible. Unless one completely overcomes all such desires, it is not possible to realise the consciousness or the soul. And without the realisation of soul or consciousness, it is not possible to connect it to God. Therefore, to connect to God, the process of Moksha or liberation, it is necessary to stop or remove the mundane desires from the mind. This process is Yoga.

There are a number of ways of developing consciousness. All are Yoga of one sort or another. They may be classified as under:

1. Jnanayoga – Attaining realisation through knowledge.
2. Karmayoga – Attaining realisation through action.
3. Bhaktiyoga – Attaining realisation through devotion.
4. Mantrayoga – Attaining realisation through Mantra (chanting litany or prayers of God).
5. Rajayoga – Attaining realisation through meditation.
6. Hathayoga – Attaining realisation through practise (physical and mental processes) and meditation.

**Hathayoga**
This is the yoga that uses force and stringent discipline in an attempt to unify the energies of the body with those of the consciousness, by using physical postures and breathing exercises. Through this method, a yogi is able to achieve considerable control over the metabolism and attain a remarkable level of physical health. Accordingly, Hathayoga employs the Asanas. Most body exercises have an effect on muscles, but the Asana have a deeper penetration power, since they not only affect muscles but also different organs and the mind. They also affect the endocrine glands, which in turn improve hormonal secretions, and hence, the various bodily functions.

Although the discipline of Hathayoga is rigorous, yet it is important to note that while practising the Asanas, the organs of body should be relaxed. There should be no stress or tension in any organ. While performing the Asanas, the breathing rate should not increase. In Yoga, there is no hurry, stress or tension at any point. This is why Yoga is the easiest way of physical and mental development, rejuvenation and prevention of diseases.

**Rajayoga**
Actually, the first four Yogas listed above, are all part of the process of Rajayoga. The word itself is derived from the Rajas

or temperament. It is the Yoga, the practice, meant for control over our individual temperament, the animalistic desire in us. Attributes of reactiveness, rage, aggressiveness, arrogance and the eternal craving of material want.

Rajayoga is Hathayoga with a difference. It is Hathayoga at a subtle level. It is the creation of natural discipline and force-flows from a deep understanding of the soul. One's soul is allowed to make attempts to achieve a desired mental posture according to whatever situation one finds oneself in. In physical Yoga, the Padmasana or the lotus posture is the most famous. A Rajyogi puts himself in this posture mentally. The soul is fixed with God in a union that is full of love, by maintaining purity of mind (lotus is the symbol of purity). Just as the roots of the lotus grow in the bed of a filthy pond but the flower is a thing of radiance and beauty, floating on the water untouched by the mud and slush, the Rajayogi lives in the material world but reaches beyond it, by maintaining a mental posture of detachment.

Bhakti is the Sanskrit term for devotion. Bhaktiyoga, then, is the yoga of devotional love. It is for those who, through loving worship of a particular deity, prophet, or saint or guru, wish to unite themselves with God. Through prayer and the faithful observation of certain rituals, the followers seek to become one with their chosen figurehead. Rajayoga involves Bhakti Yoga, in the sense, the Rajayogi's love is totally channelled in the direction of the Supreme One. Since the love is a natural one between the child (soul) and the father (Supreme Soul), there may be no need for rituals or acts of worship. The Rajayog i tries to bring in God's qualities in his practical life with total devotion or love to God. This love for God can be built on knowing Him as He is. A Rajayogi bases his love on knowledge of God.

It is important to realise that Hathayoga cannot be practised without practising Rajayoga in some form or the other. One may not give in to purely creature cravings in one's thinking and actions, while conducting procedures whose intent is the opposite. To this extent, Hathayoga may be considered an extension of Rajayoga.

# 66

# THE POWER OF PRAYER
# (NAISHTIKA TREATMENT)

Naishtika is the term employed for procedures that are supra-
natural. Paranormal phenomenon and miracles have been
known to occur and it is widely acknowledged that prayer
provides relief and inspiration to many. Sometimes a cure,
and frequently, solace and peace. The positive aspects of such
appealing, to forces that are beyond the merely human, cannot
be ignored.

The ancients classified the origins of afflictions as
*Adhyatmika* (of human or natural origin), *Adhibhoutika* (the
extraordinary or originating from malignant spirits) and
*Adhidaivika* (originating out of provocation of the
supernatural).

This led to their formulating a number of procedures to
appeal to the supernatural and to contain such forces. These
included rituals such as –

1. *Havanas* or rituals based around fire, conducted by a
   religious master of ceremonies.
2. *Yagna* or extended prayer and meditation sessions often
   employing Havanas.
3. *Bali* or sacrifice.
4. *Mantra* or reciting iitany.
5. *Japa*, such as counting prayer beads.
6. Tapa or penance.

Although benefits derived from these may be the subject of debate and investigation, there can be no doubt about the underlying principles that were behind such rituals. The principles were the adoption of –

1. Dharma
2. Karma
3. Avatara
4. Bhagavan
5. Upasana
6. Stuti
7. Pooja and prayer
8. Dhyana

All these are steps to Samadhi.
As the Geeta says:

*Samasenaiva Kaunteya Nishta Jnanasya Yapara|*
*Brahmabhuta: Prasantatma||*

When the Atma develops into the spirit of the Brahma, all affliction will be pacified.

# HERBAL CHART

| Sanskrit | Latin | English | Hindi | Gujrati | Marathi | Tamil | Telugu | Kannada | Bengali | Arabic | Pharsi |
|---|---|---|---|---|---|---|---|---|---|---|---|
| Abhaya | Terminalia Chebula | Chebulic Myrobalan | Haradh | Harade | Harade | Kandakayi | Kandookara | Alalekayi | Haseethaki | Haleelaja | Haleela |
| Agaru | Aquilaria Agalloocha | Eagle | Agar | Agar | Agar | Agali Chanada | Aguyi | — | Agaru | Ooda | — |
| Amalaki | Phylanthus Emblica | Emblica Myrobalam | Avalaa | Avala | Avalaa | Nelleekayi | Usheeroko | Nellee | Amata | — | Amlajaa |
| Ashvatta | Ficus rellegiousa | — | Peepal | Peepal | Pimpal | Arak | Ragee | Ashwatha | Ashwather amshud | Parakhel raja | Saered fig |
| Athivisha | Aconitum Heterophyllum | — | Atish | — | — | Atividayam | Atirasa | Shukla kanda — | — | — | — |
| Atibala | Sidarhambifolia | — | Kandhee | Khapaat | Mudaa | Thatee | Thuliuri Chettu | Petigu Soppu | Petari | Moshlth-ulgola | Darak-shaan |
| Badara | Zisphus Jujuba | — | Bera | Bora | Bora | Elandap | Rogavanda | Borehannu | Koola | — | — |
| Bala | Sida Cordifolia | — | Bariyar | Bal | Chikanaa | Paniyarthuti | Thelantisa | Kallangadale Bedela | Bedela | — | — |
| Bilva | Aegle-Marmelos | Bengal Quince | Baela | Baelee | Baela | Aluvigham | Baela | Baela | Baela | Saphar Jale | Beh Hindi |
| Brahmi | Herpestes Monniera | — | Pitavan | — | — | Kola | — | Kolku | Ondele | Honne | — |
| Brihatee | Solanum Indicum | — | Badee Kateri | Ubheer-inaganee | Doralee | Vyaakud | Pappara Malliee | Heggula | — | Thella Moolaka | Katayee Kalaa |
| Castor seeds | Ricinuss Comunis | — | Castor Erandi — | — | — | — | Amanakku | Amidapp-uchettu | — | — | — |

| Sanskrit | Latin | English | Hindi | Gujrati | Marathi | Tamil | Telegu | Kannada | Bengali | Arabic | Pharsi |
|---|---|---|---|---|---|---|---|---|---|---|---|
| *Chandana* | Santalum Album | Sandal-wood | Saphed Chandan | Sukhd | — | Saqndan amaram | Gandapu Chekka | Srigandha | Chandan | Sandale Abyaj | Sandala Saphed |
| *Chavya* | Piper Chaba | — | Chava | Chabak | — | — | Sevamu | Chavya | Ghavi | — | — |
| *Chitraka* | Plumbago Zeylanica | Leadwort | Cheetha | Chithro | Chitromool | Chithika | Tellachitra | Chitra Mula | Chitromool | Sheetharaj | Sheethar |
| *Dadima* | Punica Granatum | Ponia gramette | Ahar | Dadam | Dalimba | Madalayi chetti | Daninda | Dalimbe | — | Anaar | Relman |
| *Darvee* | Berbere Aristata | Indian Berberi | Daru Haladi | Daru Haldar | Daru Halad | Maramanjala | Kasturi Paspu | Kasturi Arasina | Daru Haridra | — | Dar Cotha |
| *Devadaru* | Cedrus Deodara | Deodor | Devadaru | Devadaru | Devadaru | Devadaru | Devadari | Thuppa Devadaru | Devadaru | — | — |
| *Guda* | Euphorbia Nerifolia | — | Common Milk-hedge | Guda | Sehunda | Ilayikalla | Thora | Thora | Bella | Manosa-sasing | Akuji-muchu |
| *Guggulu* | Balsamodendron Mukul | Guny Guggul | Googala | Gugal | Kamtagana | — | Gukkulu | Guggula | — | Maishakshi | Buyejah-udan |
| *Haree-Thaki* | Terminalia Chebula | — | Chebulic Myrobalan | Haradh | Harade | Harade | Kandakayi | Kandookara | Alalekayi | Haseethaki | Haleelaja Haleela |
| *Haridra* | Curcuma Longa | — | — | — | — | Haldi | Manchak | Pesupi | Arasina | — | — |
| *Jeevanthi* | Leptadenia Reticulata | — | Dodeshaka | Dodee | Khanda dakee | — | Sihi Hale | — | — | — | — |
| *Jyothishmathi* | Celestrus Paniculata | Stafftree | Italakangini | — | Mala kangoni | Balulavai | — | Jyothish-mathi | Mala kangoni | Tailan | — |
| *Kaka machi* | Solanum Nigra | Garden Night Shade | Moky | Peeludi | Komoni | Munma Thakkali | Kachipondu | Kashi Soppu | Gudaka-mayee | Inbussalab | — |

286

| Sanskrit | Latin | English | Hindi | Gujrati | Marathi | Tamil | Telugu | Kannada | Bengali | Arabic | Pharsi |
|---|---|---|---|---|---|---|---|---|---|---|---|
| *Karnanja* | — | — | Karanj | Pangam | Kamuga-chethi | Hongemera | — | — | — | — | — |
| *Karpura* | Cinnamomum Camphore | Camphor | Kapoora | Kapur | Kapoora | Karpooram | Karpooram | Karpoora | Karpoora | Kaphur | Kapoor |
| *Katuka* | Hibiscus Abelmoschus | Musk Mallow | Latha kasturi | — | Kastur babeda | Vathilai Kasturi | Kasturi | Katuka Rohini | Kala kasturi | Habbul Mushka | Mushka dana |
| *Kesara* | Crocus Sativ | Saffron | Kesara | Kesara | Kesara | Kumkum appu | Kumkuma puvva | Kumkuma Kesari | Japhraan | Japhraan | Korakee Maass |
| *Kumkuma* | — | — | — | Jafran | — | Kungo muppu | Kumkum poovu | Kesari | — | — | — |
| *Kushta* | Saussuraa Lappa | Costus | Koota | Kata | — | Koshtam | Kushtam | Kushta | Kood | Kusthe | Kushlit halkha |
| *Laksha* | Coccus Lace | Lae | Laakh | — | — | — | — | Laaksha | — | Lukh | Laakh |
| *Madana* | Randia dometarum | Emetic nut | Macirphal | Meendal | Molphal | Marukalam | Maiga | — | Madana | Jainalakai | — |
| *Madhuka* | Glycer hiza Glabra | Liquorice | Mulethi / Jeteemadhu | — | Jeshtee madh | Ati maduram | Yashti Madukan. | Jyeshta madhu | Yashti Madhu | Aslussus | — |
| *Maricha* | Piper Nigrum | Black Pepper | Kali Mirchi | — | Maree | Miree | Milagu | Miriyalu | Menasu | Golmoreech | Filfilsyah Filfilsavad |
| *Moolaka* | Raphanussativus | Radish | Mooli | Moola | Mula | Mulajee | — | Mullangi | Moolo | Phujal | Thurbi |
| *Mudga* | — | — | — | — | — | — | — | Chavya | Ghavi | — | — |
| *Musta* | Cyprus Rotundus — | — | Motha | Nagara motha | Nagara motha | Muthakaeh | Thungagan dalavim | — | Mutha | Sofrada Koophi | Mushke Jarmee |

| Sanskrit | Latin | English | Hindi | Gujrati | Marathi | Tamil | Telegu | Kannada | Bengali | Arabic | Pharsi |
|---|---|---|---|---|---|---|---|---|---|---|---|
| *Nagakesara* | Mesuaferra, (Myrica Esulenta) | — | Ironwood tree | Peela Nagakesaram | Peelam Nagakesara | Viluchampaka | — | — | Nagachem-pakam | — | Naga-kesara |
| *Nagara (Shunti)* | Zingiber Officinale | Dry Ginger | Sonta, Adrakh | Sunt | Suntee | Shukku | Sontee | Shunti | Sont | Jrnjabeela | Bekh mushkh |
| *Nirgundi* | Vitex Negundo | — | — | — | Sambalu | Vennochi-uavirti | Tella | Karilakki | — | — | — |
| *Nisha* | Curcuma Longa | Turmeric | Haldi | Haladar | Halad | Majjala | Pasupu | Arasina | Holood | Uruku saifar | Jarda choba |
| *Nyagro-dha* | Ficus Religiosa | Saened Big | Peeal | Peepalo | Pimpai | Araka | Raaii | Arali Mara | Ashudh | Shaj rathula | Darak thalarija |
| *Padma* | Nelumbium Speciosum | Saened Lotus | 'Purain | Kamala | Kamala | Tamarai | Thamaram | Kamala/Tavare | Padma | — | — |
| *Palasha* | Butea Frondosa | — | — | — | Dhak | Murukka | Moduga | Muttugamara | — | — | — |
| *Pata* | Cissampelos Pareira | Velvet leaf | Padee | Kalipat | Padaval | Appata | Pada | Agala Shunti | Akleja | — | — |
| *Patola* | Tricosanther Cocumerina | — | Paraval | Paraval | Parabal | Kamja palayi | — | Kalupa davala | Pottoal | — | — |
| *Pippali/ Pippali Moola* | Piper Longum | LongPepper | Peepal. | Peepal | Pimpalee | Tipili | Pippallu | Hippali | Pipul/ Chitramoola | Darfilfil | Filfildarj |
| *Plaksha* | Ficus Loeor | — | Pakar | Peepalee | Piparee | Pesharee | Pastari | — | — | — | — |
| *Prithveeka* | Amomum Subutem | Greater Cardamomum Elaichi | Barhi | Elactea | — | Elam | Pengu Ellakkaylu | Elakki | Badetach | Kakule | Heela kaala |
| *Pudina* | Mentha Viridis | Spearmint | Pudeena | Phudino | Pudeena | Pudeena | Pudeena | Pudeena | Pudeena | Phoodanja | Poodin |
| *Punarnava* | — | — | — | Biskapara | Sukuyetti | Galijeru | | Kommeberu | | | |

| Sanskrit | Latin | English | Hindi | Gujrati | Marathi | Tamil | Telegu | Kannada | Bengali | Arabic | Pharsi |
|---|---|---|---|---|---|---|---|---|---|---|---|
| *Raktaveshta* | Rubia Cordifolia | Indian Madder | Manjeet | Majeeta | Manjista | Mandita | Tamra-Vallee | Raktha Manjista | Mnjister | Phulba | Runasa |
| *Sariva* | Hemidesmus Indicus | Indian Sarsaparilla | Anantha Mcola | Uparsalee | Uparsal | Nannari | Muktha pulagam | Namada Beru | Kapuri | — | — |
| *Sarshapa seed* | Brassica Campestris | — | — | Sarso | — | Kadagu | Sasuvalu | Sasive | Sasuvalu | — | — |
| *Sarshapathaila* | Brassica Alba | Rape (seed) | Sarson | Sarasav | Shirasee | — | Avalu | Sasuve | Shorshey | Huort Abyaru | Sarshapa |
| *Shathavri* | Asparagus Racemosa | Wild Asparagus | Sathavar | Sathavar | Sathavari | Sadavar | Chatta | Ashadi Beru | — | — | — |
| *Snuhi* | Euphorbia Nerifolia | — | — | — | Thuhar | Elaikalli | Akuchi-mudu | Muru Enikalli | — | — | — |
| *Sookshmaela* | Elettaria Cardomum | Lesser Cardomum | Chhoti Ilaichi | Choth Elagh | Belachee | Illayi | Illayee | Elakki | Choto Elaach | Kakul | Heelvaka |
| *Surbali* | PinusLongifolia | Long-leaved Pine | Cheedh | Teliyo Devadar | — | Sarala-devadaru | Devadaru Chettu | Thuppa Devadaru | — | — | — |
| *Tagara* | Valeriana Wallichi | Indian Valerian | Thagara | Thagara Gamtoda | Nagar mool | — | — | Sugandha Bala | Mushkaval | — | Asaaroon |
| *Talisa* | Abies Webbiana | — | — | — | Talispatra | Talispatra | Talispatralu | Talispatre | — | — | — |
| *Thambula* | Piper Betel | Betalvine | Pan | nagarvel | Nagvela | Vethilai | Thampa lapaku | Viledele | Paan | Thambool | Thambool |
| *Thuvaraka* | Hydrocarpus Wightiana | — | Chala Mogara | Papitha | Kudaka veeta | Maravathayi | Adais Badamu | Garuda Phala | Choul Mugara | — | Biranj Megara |
| *Tila* | Sesamum Indicum | Sesamum | Thila | Thala | Thil | Ellu | Gubbulu | Ellu | Thila | Samsam | Kunjad |

| Sanskrit | Latin | English | Hindi | Gujrati | Marathi | Tamil | Telegu | Kannada | Bengali | Arabic | Pharsi |
|---|---|---|---|---|---|---|---|---|---|---|---|
| **Twak** | Cinnamomum Zeylanica | Cinnamon | Dalchini | Dalchini | Kuruya | Thaja | Thaja | Dalchini | Dalchini | Sanalifu | Darchin |
| **Ushna** | Zingiber Officinale | Dry Ginger | Sonta, Adrakh | Sunt | Suntee | Shukku | Sontee | Shunti | Sont | Jrnjabeela | Bekh mushkh |
| **Usira** | Andropogon | Squarrosus | Khus | Elamache | Vetlivera | Lamancha | — | — | — | — | — |
| **Uthpala** | Nymphoea Stellata | Indian Water Lily | Kuyee | Poyanu | Kamoda | Nalla kalava | Allikada | Uthpala | Shamglic | — | Neelofer |
| **Vasa** | Adhatoda Vasica | — | — | Aduba | — | Adodirlayi | Adasaram | Adusoge | — | — | — |
| **Vibheethaki** | Terminalia Belerica | Beleric Myrobalam | Baheda | Baheda | Vayadaa | Akkam | Thadi | Tharekayi | Baheda | Baleela | Balleelaja |
| **Vidanga** | Embelia Ribes | — | Bhabeeranga | Vavdeeng | Vavding | Vayu Vilamagam | Vayu Vilamagam | Vayu Vidanga | — | — | — |
| **Vidari** | Puraria Tuberose | — | Vidarikanda | Khaakhar vela | Bedariya bela | — | — | — | Shemida | — | — |
| **Vyaghree** | Solamum Xanthocarpum | Wild Eggplant | Chitkateri | Boyrin gatice | Bhuyeer ingance | Kandam Kantiri | Koodaa | Nellagulla | Kantikuari | Badam Jambaree | Badam Gambaree |
| **Yashti Madhu** | Glycerhiza Glabra | Liquorice | Mulethi Jeteemadhu | — | Jeshtee madh | Atimaduram Yashti Madukam | Yashti Madukam | Jyeshta madhu | Yashti Madhu | Aslussus | — |

# BIBLIOGRAPHY

1. Angaranga - Kalyanamalla
2. Atharva Veda
3. Balatantra Streerogadhikara - Kalyanamalla 34
4. Bhavaprakasha Madhyama Khanda-Yoni Rogadhikara 33
5. Bhishajya Ratnavali Streeroga Yoni Vyapat Chikitsa 3, 9 & 41
6. Brihat Yoga Tarangini 41
7. Charaka Chikitsa Sthana
8. Charaka Chikitsa, chapter 1 (Padas 1,2,3 & 4), chapter 2 (Pada 1), chapters 4 & 8
9. Charaka Nidana, chapter 6
10. Charaka Samhita Sutrsthana, chapters 5, 7, 8, 9, 10, 11, 16, 17, 18, 21, 25, 26, 28, & 30
11. Charaka Shareera, chapters 1, 3, 4, 5, 6 & 8
12. Charaka Siddhi, chapters 11 & 12
13. Charaka Vimana, chapters 1, 2, 3, 6, & 8
14. Devaraj, Dr. T.L.; Ayurveda for Health & Family Welfare
15. Devaraj, Dr. T.L.; Ayurveda for Healthy Living
16. Devaraj, Dr. T.L.; The Panchakarma Treatment of Ayurveda
17. Devaraj, Dr. T.L.; "Family Planning in Ayurvedic System of Medicine"; the magazine of Government College of Indian Medicine

291

18. Dhyani, Dr. S.S. ; Yoga and Ayurveda

19. Gala Dr. D.R. & others; Juice Diet for Perfect Health

20. Gala Dr. D.R. & others; Nature Cure for Every Disease

21. Human Physiology by Chatterjee

22. Indian Journal of the History of Sciences, Number 1

23. Iyengar, Sri B.K.S.; Yogadeepika

24. Keshava Murthy, H.S.; Yoga Treatment (in Kannada)

25. Manusmriti, chapters 2, 3, 4, 5, 6, 12 & 14

26. Mahabharata (Shanti Parva), chapters 59 & 90

27. Mysore Gazetteer June 1930 : Establishment of Birth
Control Clinics in the Victoria & Maternity Hospitals of
Bangalore and Mysore

28. Nature Cure Treatment : Institute of Naturopathy and Yogic
Sciences (in Kannada)

29. Panasyaka, chapters 3 & 85

30. Pandit Laxmi Doss; Meditation for Everybody

31. Patanjali Yogasutra

32. Raman B.V.; Astrological Magazine 5,6 & 21 of 1967

33. Rasa Ratna Samuchaya, chapters 9 & 26

34. Rasaprakasha Sudhakara Yeshodara

35. Rati Manjari

36. Rati Rashaya Kokkada Kuchimara Tantra

37. Roy, Meera; Brihataranya Upanishat and Atharvanaveda

38. Subhashita Tarangini

39. Sushruta Chikitsa, chapters 24 & 25

40. Sushruta Samhita Sutra, chapters 1, 5 & 15

41. Sushruta Shareera, chapter 10

42. Vivekananda Yoga Kendra, Bangalore (in Kannada)

43. Yogaratnakara

44. Jindal, I.N.Y.S.; Nature Cure: A Way of Life